OXFORD SPECIALTY TRAINING

The MRCPCH Clinical Exam Made Simple

T0177782

OXFORD SPECIALTY TRAINING

The MRCPCH Clinical Exam Made Simple

Dr Stanley Tamuka Zengeya
MB ChB, MRCP (UK), MMeD (Paeds), MSc, FRCPCH
Consultant Paediatrician, Great Western Hospitals NHS Foundation Trust, Swindon
Honorary Senior Lecturer, University of Bristol
Clinical Professor, University of St. George's Medical School, Grenada

Dr Tiroumourougane Serane V
MB BS, MRCPCH (UK), MD Paed., DNB Paed., MNAMS
Associate Professor, Department of Paediatrics, Sri Lakshmi Narayana Institute of Medical Sciences,
Puducherry, India
Formerly Clinical Fellow in Paediatrics and Neonatology, Great Western Hospital, Swindon

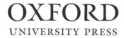
OXFORD
UNIVERSITY PRESS

OXFORD
UNIVERSITY PRESS

Great Clarendon Street, Oxford OX2 6DP

Oxford University Press is a department of the University of Oxford.
It furthers the University's objective of excellence in research, scholarship,
and education by publishing worldwide in

Oxford New York

Auckland Cape Town Dar es Salaam Hong Kong Karachi
Kuala Lumpur Madrid Melbourne Mexico City Nairobi
New Delhi Shanghai Taipei Toronto

With offices in
Argentina Austria Brazil Chile Czech Republic France Greece
Guatemala Hungary Italy Japan Poland Portugal Singapore
South Korea Switzerland Thailand Turkey Ukraine Vietnam

Oxford is a registered trade mark of Oxford University Press
in the UK and in certain other countries

Published in the United States
by Oxford University Press Inc., New York

British Library Cataloguing in Publication Data
Data available

Library of Congress Cataloging in Publication Data
Data available

Typeset in GillSans by Cenveo, Bangalore, India
Printed in Great Britain
on acid-free paper by
CPI Antony Rowe, Chippenham, Wiltshire

ISBN 978–0–19–958793–3

10 9 8 7

Printed and bound in Great Britian by Ashford Colour Press Ltd, Gosport, Hants.

We dedicate this book to our parents
Mr Tarutora Miles Zengeya and Mrs Jessie Zengeya, and
Mr Vidjayarangane Serane A and Mrs Canagammalle.

Foreword

The Membership Examination of the Royal College of Paediatrics and Child Health (MRCPCH) has undergone considerable changes in the last few years. The aim has been to make the content and the process of the examination transparent and fit for the purpose of correctly identifying competency amongst trainees embarking on specialty training in paediatrics.

Although the College Examination Committee has done an excellent job in bringing about the quite major changes to the exam that were needed, there is still a potential gap between what experienced examiners expect in the clinical examination and the way trainees have gained their experience.

Not surprisingly, there are still doctors who genuinely do not understand why they have failed the examination after all the hard work they have put into their preparations. The unique aspects of paediatric practice, which make history taking and examination of children with their parents such a challenge to any doctor, can be particularly stressful to trainees at this stage of their career.

A multimedia DVD cannot substitute for clinical experience with real patients, but is a valuable way of illustrating and commenting on very particular issues, which are often taken for granted in the busy clinic situation.

Dr Zengeya and Dr Serane and their colleagues have done an excellent job in emphasizing the need for candidates to concentrate on the precise objective of each examination station. They need to understand the expectations of the examiners and to follow precisely the instructions they are given. As well as a structured approach to demonstrating their skills, candidates must be able to show they have the ability to present their findings concisely, with confidence and a lack of ambiguity. The time constraints of each examination station must be understood. This can be challenging, and so practice is invaluable.

The editors are to be congratulated and thanked for the high standard of this production, which will be of invaluable assistance to MRCPCH examination candidates. Close attention to both the verbal and non-verbal content will repay the candidate well in preparation for this step into the most rewarding of specialities in medicine.

I wish you all good luck, both in the exam and in your future careers.

Andrew Wilkinson

Andrew Wilkinson
Professor of Paediatrics, Oxford

Preface

The MRCPCH clinical exam is the most important hurdle any paediatric trainee must leap in their path to become a fully-fledged paediatrician. The exam format changed a few years ago with the emphasis shifting from short and long cases to the more modern, system-based Objective Structured Clinical Examination (OSCE). The examination is now primarily competency based, where the candidates are expected to show how they would handle a clinical problem which they would face in real-life situations in a controlled environment. Additional emphasis has been placed on communication skills, with two stations included to evaluate the candidate's skills in this area.

To pass the exam, candidates are expected to be efficient, clear, and to demonstrate a structured examination technique. Although many clinical books are available on paediatric examination, there is a shortage of teaching material preparing candidates for this exam. This book and accompanying DVD have been produced to fill this void.

In this book, we aim to show the candidate an acceptable approach to examining a child in an exam setting. The principles of examination of various cases are outlined and a framework is provided, which will help the candidate achieve the expected standard. Emphasis has been placed on commonly neglected topics such as focused history taking, effective communication, and preparation for the exam. This book teaches the candidate to **focus on the child** and uses the same format for all systems. The simple, concise, yet comprehensive approach should make for easy reading, and the line drawings and photographs are visually appealing. We have made a conscious effort to avoid exhaustive theory, which can be read in depth in various textbooks of paediatrics.

A unique aspect of this project is that experienced paediatricians and examiners have stepped into the role of the candidate and demonstrated the clinical skills required to pass various stations. They demonstrate a structured approach to the various systems in the allotted time, which gives prospective candidates an opportunity to observe, listen, and learn. The videos show the candidate how to make the clinical examination fun and interesting for the child by establishing rapport with them and putting them at ease. The videos teach the candidates skills that are difficult to convey in a written form. The videos are a visual aid, consolidating the adage 'If you tell me, I will forget, if you show me I will remember'. In addition, the DVD also contains 'live candidates' taking a mock exam, with examiners giving comments (both positive and negative) about their performance. This will appeal to prospective candidates as it will help them to avoid some of the pitfalls that are highlighted.

In conclusion, this book and accompanying DVD are designed to simplify the preparation for the MRCPCH clinical exam. After reading it and watching the videos, candidates should be able to practise on their own and reach the expected standard. Practice makes perfect!

Video

Video 0.1 Drs Serane and Zengeya give introductory remarks.

Acknowledgements

Producing this book and the DVD required a huge team effort from various individuals and experts. We thank all those who worked tirelessly to make this project a success and to whom we are ever so grateful. We thank Lyn Hill-Tout, the Chief Executive at the Great Western Hospitals NHS Foundation Trust, and the Medical Director, Dr Alf Troughton, who allowed this project to take place at the Great Western Hospitals NHS Foundation Trust, where the clinical station videos were filmed. We extend our special thanks and gratitude to the children and their families who took part in the filming of videos. We thank all the contributors who shared their knowledge, experience, and time in this project. The contributors included a strong team of experienced medical professionals, MRCPCH Examiners, Hospital Consultants, Specialist Registrars, junior medical staff, and patients. These contributors are too many to mention by name. Our special thanks to Professor Andrew Wilkinson, Dr Nick Archer, and all our paediatric consultant colleagues at the Great Western Hospital, Dr Janet King, Dr Paul O'Keeffe, Dr Helen Price, Dr Ravi Chinthapalli, and Dr Lyn Williamson, who helped us in this task. We thank Dr Anna Kilonback for helping with some of the clinical examination photographs. We thank Nhlanhla Sibanda and M&N Video Productions for filming the clinical stations.

We thank our families for their sacrifice during the time we were writing the book and filming the videos. Our wives Anna Zengeya (Stanley) and Bhuvaneswari (Tiroumourougane) deserve special mention for their great sacrifice during the long, arduous process of completing this project. We thank our children for giving up some of their time and the interaction we cherish. Without their support we could not have achieved this task. We would like to acknowledge the support provided by Christopher Read and Katy Loftus of OUP.

Video

Video 0.2 Acknowledgements.

Contents

Contributors

Dr Nick Archer MA, MB BChir FRCP FRCPCH DCH
Consultant Paediatric Cardiologist, Oxford Children's Hospital
Honorary Clinical Senior Lecturer, University of Oxford
(Contributed parts of chapter 5)

Dr Paul Timothy O'Keeffe MB BS, BSc, MRCP (UK), MRCPCH
Consultant Paediatrician, Great Western Hospitals NHS Foundation Trust, Swindon
(Contributed parts of chapter 13)

Dr Lyn Williamson BM BCh, MA (Oxon), DRCOG, DCH, MRCGP, FRCP
Consultant Rheumatologist, Great Western Hospitals NHS Foundation Trust, Swindon
Honorary Senior Lecturer, University of Oxford
(Contributed parts of chapter 12)

Contributors to the DVD

Dr Nick Archer MA, MB, BChir, FRCP, FRCPCH, DCH
Consultant Paediatric Cardiologist, Oxford Children's Hospital
Honorary Clinical Senior Lecturer, University of Oxford

Dr Ravindranath Chinthapalli MB BS, DCH, MRCP (UK), FRCPCH
Consultant Paediatrician, Great Western Hospitals NHS Foundation Trust, Swindon

Dr Sri Dantuluri MBBS, MD, MRCPCH
Specialist Registrar in Hepatology, Leeds

Dr Karen Jenkins MRCGP
GP Partner, Nottingham

Dr Akhila Kavirayani MBBS, MD Paediatrics, MRCPCH
Specialist Registrar in Paediatrics, Bristol Royal Hospital for Children

Dr Janet King MB, FRCP, FRCPCH
Consultant Paediatrician, Great Western Hospitals NHS Foundation Trust, Swindon
Honorary Senior Lecturer, University of Bristol

Dr Paul Timothy O'Keeffe MB BS, BSc, MRCP (UK), MRCPCH
Consultant Paediatrician, Great Western Hospitals NHS Foundation Trust, Swindon

Dr Helen Price MD, FAAP, FRCPCH
Consultant Paediatrician, Great Western Hospitals NHS Foundation Trust, Swindon

Dr Angus Tallini MRCS, MRCGP
GP Principal, Falkland Surgery, Newbury, Berkshire

Chapter 1 **How to prepare for the MRCPCH clinical examination**

About the clinical examination

The clinical examination for the MRCPCH is a major hurdle that every aspiring paediatrician has to face in their career. As the exam is designed to differentiate between the prepared and unprepared candidates, it is important to be well trained. To pass the MRCPCH exam, the candidate needs to demonstrate that they have the clinical skills expected of a newly appointed specialist registrar. According to the Royal College of Paediatrics and Child Health, the aim of the examination is to 'improve the standard of medical care, educate and examine doctors and provide information to the public on the health care of children'. Competence is expected in various aspects of paediatric medicine, including history taking, communication, establishment of rapport, physical examination, clinical judgement, professional behaviour, and ethical practice. On the Royal College of Paediatrics and Child Health website, www.rcpch.ac.uk, a lot of information is provided for candidates. Every candidate is encouraged to visit this website before sitting the exam.

Conventionally, the MRCPCH clinical exam consisted of a long case, a short cases, and a viva. However, concerns were raised about the validity of the traditional system, as it focused mainly on knowledge rather than competence. According to George Miller, who proposed a pyramidal framework for assessing clinical competence, the lowest level of the pyramid of assessment is the evaluation of knowledge. This is tested by written examinations. At the second level, the assessment tests not only the theoretical knowledge but also the application of this knowledge. At the third level, the individual has knowledge, knows how to do it, and shows how it is done. This is the level of 'true competence' and the MRCPCH clinical examination tests at this level (figure 1.1). In 2004, a major change was brought about in the clinical examination, in which competency-based 'objective structured clinical examination' replaced the traditional system. In the new MRCPCH clinical examination, the candidate goes through a 'circuit' of clinical stations. Competency-based assessments provide a measure of the subject's skills in controlled representations of clinical practice and are regarded by both candidates and examiners as a fairer evaluation method. Candidates are given instructions either by the examiner or in written format with a predetermined 'opening statement'. The current format tests several key areas that are considered to be essential for a competent clinician. These skills include communication, systematic and directed clinical examination, developmental assessment, logical organization of thoughts, and management planning.

The MRCPCH clinical exam measures the extent of the learner's knowledge, skills, and attitudes, to determine the success or failure of the candidate. This is chiefly a *skill-based examination and is a critical test of the candidate's bedside behaviour and diagnostic competence*. The examiners are *not looking for encyclopaedic knowledge*; they are just looking to ascertain that the candidate can be trusted to carry out a satisfactory clinical examination, make competent assessments, and formulate an appropriate management plan. In essence, the examiner wants to know whether the candidate would be safe and competent as a registrar working in a busy unit.

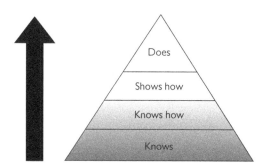

Figure 1.1 A simple model of competence.

From: Miller GE. The assessment of clinical skills/ performance. *Acad Med* 1990: **65** (Suppl.); S63–67.

It is important to attempt the exam only when both the aspirant and the supervisor feel the candidate is ready. The clinical exam is divided into ten OSCE-style (Objective Structured Clinical Examination) stations, covering a wide range of systems and scenarios. The candidate should be fully acquainted with the exam circuit, as lack of knowledge of the exam format may lead to failure (figure 1.2). Like any other assessment, it is important to understand not only the format, but also the objectives of each of the components. By a better understanding of what is being assessed, preparation (and practise) can be geared along those lines. The College has prepared 'anchor' statements outlining criteria to grade the performances for each station. They provide examiners with guidance for marking the performance of the candidate. Examiners are paired up at the start of each circuit to set standards for awarding marks. These standards enable a decision to be made on what constitutes a pass, fail, clear pass, or clear fail and will be sent with the candidates' exam sheets to the college for future reference. Examiners also agree on what they regard as an appropriate 'opening statement' for each station, which will be used for every candidate passing through that station. It is important for candidates to listen carefully to this statement.

The candidate should focus only on the current station without worrying about the previous ones. The examiners do not know what has gone on in the stations before, which removes any bias from poor performance in the preceding stations. Candidates are marked according to their performance in the broad categories of conduct, examination skills, and discussion with the examiner. In the category of conduct, marks are awarded for professional behaviour, ability to establish rapport, putting the child at ease, and communication skills with both the child and the parents. In the category of examination skills, evaluation is based on the candidate's ability to perform the clinical examination in a structured fluent way, to identify and interpret the clinical signs accurately. Finally, marks are also given to the candidate for their ability to discuss the differential diagnoses and management plan. Marks are awarded as clear pass (12), pass (10), bare fail (8), clear fail (4), and unacceptable (0). To pass the exam the candidate has to score 100 marks. The candidate must pass in every section to gain an overall pass. If a candidate achieves a bare fail in one station, they may be able to compensate for this by scoring a clear pass in another station. Candidates who score poorly are advised to defer retaking the exam for one (marks between 70 and 80) or two sittings (marks below 70).

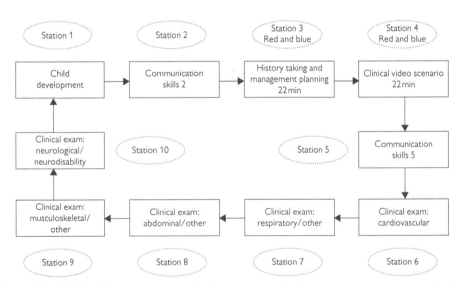

Figure 1.2 MRCPCH clinical examination circuit. All stations are of 9 minutes' duration, except stations 3 and 4 which are each 22 minutes in length.

From the Royal College of Paediatrics web site, www.rcpch.ac.uk.

How to prepare

These suggestions may appear didactic in nature but, obviously, it depends on the individual!

> Learn to see, learn to hear, learn to feel, learn to smell and know that by practice alone can you become expert. Medicine is learned at the bedside and not in the classroom.
>
> *Sir William Osler, 1919*

In the clinical exam, your skills rather than theoretical knowledge are tested. The examiner's intention is to gain a reflection of the candidate's clinical competence. The competent candidate will identify relevant clinical signs and coherently give an account of the findings in a professional manner. Most of the preparation should be at the bedside with patients, as clinical competence cannot be gained from textbooks. However, it is essential to learn the correct clinical methods from books and consultants and then practise repeatedly until you perfect the methods. Clinical skills can be acquired only through thoughtful preparation, reflection, and purposeful practice. Incorporating the newly gained skills in day-to-day practice makes it easier to use them in the examination.

Physical preparation

For success in the exam, mere academic and mental preparation is not sufficient. When preparing for exams, preserving physical well-being is as important as mental preparation. As the common phrase 'A sound mind in a sound body' says, you need complete physical and mental well-being. Tiredness, poor nutrition, and stimulants undermine performance in the exam.

- Keep your life as balanced as possible, especially during exam time.
- As far as possible, eat and sleep properly and regularly. Go to bed and get up at the same time each day.
- Eat a balanced, healthy diet.
- Limit your alcohol intake.
- Cut down on caffeine intake.

Mental preparation

- For many of us, studying can be hard work. Many people regard exam preparation as one of the most professionally rewarding challenges of their career.
- Reinforce positive thinking. Believe in yourself, that you can succeed because you have the ability and have prepared perfectly.
- Avoid those who seem worried or scared about the exam, as they can negatively affect your composure.
- Cultivate equanimity, which is the controlling of emotional or mental agitation by will or as a matter of habit even under hostile conditions.

Emotional preparation

Often, exams cause severe anxiety. You should therefore have a plan in place to deal with it in the exam setting.
- Use positive self-talk, and focus on what you will do next in the exam.
- Practise relaxation techniques such as meditation or deep breathing. This will help to calm your frayed nerves and settle you down. It will also help you to focus and gather your thoughts.

More than six months before the exam

- Improve your knowledge in paediatrics by going through a standard textbook of paediatrics and study the 'how to treat', 'education and practice', photographs, and clinical guideline sections of paediatric journals such as the *Archives of Disease of Childhood*.

- Study information on all the common diseases, though not in great detail.
- Prepare yourself by gathering sufficient core knowledge of any condition you see in a patient.
- Read material from websites such as the Department of Health (www.dh.gov.uk), National Institute for Health and Clinical Excellence (www.nice.org.uk), NHS Clinical Knowledge Summaries (www.cks.nhs.uk), Scottish Intercollegiate Guidelines Network (www.sign.ac.uk), and NHS Evidence Health Information Resources (www.library.nhs.uk), which provide policies, guidance, and information on various childhood conditions.

One to six months before the exam

- Collect all the resource materials with which you are planning to prepare.
- Set a start date for preparation and a study timetable. Leave the last few weeks for revision.
- Speak to past candidates, whose experience of the list of topics can be useful.
- Plan your study leave and the 'off duty' days, both for the exam and any courses you may wish to attend.
- Form a study group:
  - Find others who are planning to sit the exam at the same time and form a small group of about four to six people.
  - Meet regularly, discuss, and practise clinical examinations.
  - Get one person to play the role of the patient, one doing the task, and (if possible) one watching, timing, and commenting on the technique using a sample mark sheet. In doing this, you will be able to get a feel for running to time and working under pressure.
- Advantages of preparing in a study group:
  - Sharing of information about resources and interesting cases is useful.
  - It is an opportunity to practise clinical scenarios and examinations.
  - Presenting cases and teaching one another cements your learning.
- While preparing:
  - Be familiar with core content and orient to key concepts of the clinical examination.
  - Prioritize your reading and learn to focus on clinical conditions you often encounter.
  - Work out an examination approach for each system that suits you; practise this over and over until it is second nature to you; these steps should become part of routine examination in your clinical practice.
  - Practise your presentation style; be concise but clear; rank the patient's problems; focus on the main points, differential diagnosis, and management plan. Remember, examiners like candidates to be polished and thorough.
  - Consider all the cases in your routine practice as if they were your exam cases and approach them in a similar manner to the exam.
  - Ask your registrars, colleagues, and consultants to assess and give feedback on your performance.
  - Organize regular teaching sessions by the consultants or registrars in your wards. Visits to teaching hospitals for clinical teaching might be useful for those in district general hospitals.
  - Take the time to visit the specialist wards—cardiology, respiratory medicine, neurology, rheumatology, dermatology, developmental assessment units—and gain as much exposure as possible.
- Learn to answer to the point. If the examiner asks 'What is the diagnosis?' you should say it immediately and give the reasons based on your clinical findings, for example 'The diagnosis is Down's syndrome based on the following features', and then list them. State the most important findings first. Give both the positive and negative findings.

- Learn to summarize. Try the four-point presentation:
  1. General findings: 'On examination the patient looks comfortable and he is small for his age. I would like to plot his age and height on a centile chart'.
  2. Important positive findings: 'My main findings were jaundice and an enlarged liver 3 cm below the costal margin which was hard but smooth'.
  3. Important negative findings: 'However, there were no ascites or dilated veins on the abdomen'.
  4. Clinical conclusion: 'These findings would be consistent with biliary atresia'.
- Attend a clinical course for the membership exam if possible.

The week before the exam

- Arrange a simulated examination practice with a 'mock' examiner (consultant, experienced registrar, or fellow trainee). Arrange these with different people to broaden your experience and learn how to respond to the varied approaches of different examiners.
- Practise the timing of the clinical cases in your study group and get used to the pace of the exam.
- Do more and more physical examinations on 'real patients'.
- When you are nervous and stressed, take some time out and relax before restarting your preparation.

On the day of the exam

- Obviously, the clinical exam will be a stressful experience and so make sure you are well rested the night before the exam.
- Be positive that you will have a successful exam.
- Dress conservatively to convey professionalism.
  - Men can wear a suit with a tie. Avoid the white coat! Do not forget to carry a watch. Carry a comb for a last-minute touch-up. Fingernails should be short. Shoes should be comfortable with socks that match the shoes.
  - Women can wear a trouser suit or knee-length skirt, minimal conservative style jewellery, and make-up. Have neat, non-fussy hair, which should be kept out of your face. Avoid using heavy perfumes. Fingernails should be short, ideally without polish, or with neutral colour only. Shoes should be comfortable, preferably without high heels. Carry a comb or brush for a last-minute touch-up.
- Organize material (identity document, admission letter, equipment such as stethoscope, toy, patella hammer, ophthalmoscope, measuring tape, alcohol gel) the day before the exam. However, remember that all the equipment you need, except a stethoscope, might be in the room and so look around and see what is there and use it if appropriate!
- Arrive early so that you have the time to prepare mentally and analyse the exam situation.

During the exam

- Smile! Be calm and confident. Fear is fine, but keep it in your heart and not on your face or in your handshake. *After all, it is an exam and, even if you do not triumph, you will learn new things which will help you to succeed later.* Do not adopt the attitude that this is a difficult examination and everybody fails it.
- Adopt a good bedside manner, including a good approach to the patient, referring to the patient by their 'correct' name, and obtaining consent before physical examination.
- Look professional and show that you have done this many times before. Remember, *do not hesitate anywhere*. Proceed as if you are confident about what you are doing.

- Ensure the patient is as comfortable as possible. Expose the area for examination without overexposure or underexposure. Remember to keep the patient warm always.
- Follow infection control measures such as hand washing or decontaminating with alcohol gel.
- Speak slowly and clearly and make eye contact with the examiner.
- Be sensitive to the needs of the child throughout the assessment.
- Remember, if you are talking in front of the patient avoid using words that are likely to alarm or upset the patient and the family, such as cancer or cerebral palsy. Instead, use euphemisms such as neoplastic disease or developmental delay.
- Be meticulous in your approach and complete the examination in every station. Examine everything even if it seems irrelevant.
- Describe your findings clearly before you make a diagnosis. State important positives and negatives.
- *Always be honest.* Do not make up physical signs or give conflicting findings. Think carefully about what you want to say before you speak. If you have made an error, retract the remark and start again.
- Often, the examiner may prompt you to bring you back on track if you are straying from what they want, so listen carefully to the examiner.
- However, do not expect encouragement or feedback from the examiner! This is an assessment and not a teaching session. A positive atmosphere is not necessarily a guide to passing or failing. Ignore the atmosphere and concentrate on what the examiner asks you to do.
- *Don't argue* your case too strongly with the examiner. Do only what the examiners ask you to do. Don't mess around as this will irritate the examiner. If you feel the examiner is leading you to reconsider your diagnosis, be prepared and keep an open mind.
- Do not be overconfident! Humility is a good virtue.
- Try to keep your answers as direct and brief as possible. If you stretch your answers unnecessarily, it is possible the examiner will come up with new questions out of your answers.
- You can influence what discussion might follow by what you say. If you are not sure about something, do not mention it. Avoid long periods of silence! Keep talking whenever possible.
- Stay calm even when you are not sure of the diagnosis. Focus on the clinical findings and not on the diagnosis. Offer a differential diagnosis and management plan. If you are not sure of the diagnosis, give a differential diagnosis first. If you know the diagnosis, say it!
- Do not rush your presentation and risk missing important points.
- Do not allow the examiner's facial expression or mannerism to put you off. Some examiners are 'hawks', which may make you feel that you are doing badly. Some examiners are 'doves', acting benignly, which might lure you into a false sense that you are doing well. Keep your focus and ignore any distractions.
- Do not be distracted by real or imaginary mistakes from previous stations. Remember, a few minor mistakes will not make you fail. The examiners in each station are not aware of your performance in the previous station. Even if you have made some errors, press on with the task at hand. Do not convince yourself that you are doing badly. Dispirited candidates perform progressively worse and may give up before completing the examination.
- Do not assume that behind every case, there is a trap or rare diagnosis which you have never come across. Most of the cases and questions are straightforward and need simple answers.
- Don't try to be clever. Give simple answers to simple questions.
- Never think you have failed until you get your result.

You CAN and WILL pass this exam!

Chapter 2 **Effective communication in the exam**

Communication is not just giving information; rather, it is a two-way process and involves the exchange of information, ideas, and knowledge. Effective communication is the key to success and can be achieved only if the receiver understands the exact information the sender is aiming to transfer. Medical communication is the art of speaking clearly and professionally, while reducing the possibility of being misunderstood. It will increase patient satisfaction and trust and improve understanding of treatment and compliance. Examiners consider effective communication to be the most essential skill any doctor requires to deal with the patient's problems. The General Medical Council has highlighted the importance of communicating well by stating that 'medical graduates must be able to communicate clearly, sensitively and effectively, not only with patients and their relatives, but also with colleagues and other healthcare professionals'.

The Royal College of Paediatrics and Child Heath has put so much emphasis on communication that this is the only skill that is tested in two independent stations in the clinical examination. The College feels that a careful assessment of communication skills distinguishes the good candidates from the bad ones. Often, overseas-trained candidates and non-native English speakers find this station difficult, as they may not have grasped the basic skills of this assessment. In this station, the examiner will watch a communication scenario between the candidate and the patient's family. It is of utmost importance to read the instructions carefully and understand them. A common mistake is to confuse this station with history taking. The examiner's task is to observe only and not to ask any questions or make any comments on the candidate's performance. At the end of the episode, the examiner will evaluate the candidate's performance. The key competence skills required in the communication station are given in table 2.1.

Effective communication—the theory

Effective communication is a two-way process in which there is an **exchange of thoughts, feelings, or ideas** towards a mutually accepted goal. **Speaking and listening** are the two arms of

Table 2.1 Key competence skills required in the communication station

Competence skill	Standard
To understand the process of communicating with children and their families	Show appropriate skills in the triadic consultation: child, family and doctor
To understand how to communicate with a child	Understand the importance of age in communicating with a child
	Engage the child during conversation and use suitable language which the child can understand
To demonstrate competence in asking questions	Employ both open and closed questions in communication
	Show proper wording of open-ended and directed questions and correct use of each type of question
Awareness of communicating effectively and sensitively	Capacity to communicate effectively in a time-limited scenario
	Demonstrate the ability to address relevant issues
	Avoid getting superficial and superfluous information irrelevant to the main problem
Understand the various elements of effective communication	Display the ability to use verbal and non-verbal cues in communication
	Demonstrate the ability to listen to the family or child and show empathy
	Show awareness of the need to check the patient's or parent's understanding and answer any questions raised
Competence in summarizing the information	Summarize the information discussed
	Offer more support to the family and opportunities in future for further discussion

effective communication. One cannot be an effective communicator if both speaking and listening are not mastered.

Medical communication starts with speaking, which requires **a sender, a message, a medium or channel, and a receiver**. The sender encodes a package of information and transmits this by a medium to the receiver. Commonly used media include air, noise, signal, and paper. Content and context are the two elements of information that will be transmitted via the medium. **Content** is the actual words or symbols. **Context** is the way the message is delivered, that is the non-verbal components such as body language, facial expressions, posture, gestures, eye contact, and state of emotion. During communication, context is extremely important as it helps the patient and the doctor to understand one another. On receiving the message, the recipient decodes it and can give the sender **feedback** (figure 2.1).

Context has static and dynamic components. The static components are distance, orientation, posture, and physical contact. The distance between the speaker and recipient reflects the intensity of the exchange. In general, it should be about an arm's length without any intervening object such as a table. **Posture** conveys the interest in the conversation and the best posture is sitting upright, leaning forward slightly with the arms open. Physical contact such as shaking hands, touching, or patting on the back reflects an element of intimacy and is useful to convey empathy.

Facial expressions, gestures, eye contact, and vocal elements are some of the dynamic components of context. Facial expressions such as smile, frown, raised eyebrow, yawn, and sneer convey interest or the lack of it and are watched constantly by the recipient. Gestures are hand movements, which can express the speaker's intent and interest. Eye contact is a principal feature of communication and can convey emotion, reluctance, interest, or boredom. Failure to maintain eye contact may suggest depression, embarrassment, or lack of interest in the conversation. Excessive eye contact may point to anger or aggression. Vocal elements such as tone, pitch, rhythm, and loudness signal various emotions.

Feedback helps to convey the recipient's understanding to the speaker and can be either verbal or non-verbal (e.g. nodding the head to show agreement). Providing feedback is not repeating the speaker's words; rather, it is expressing the meaning using different words to achieve greater clarity.

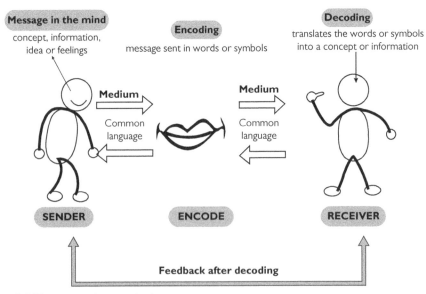

Figure 2.1 The process of communication.

Active listening is the foundation of effective communication. While hearing is the act of reception of sound, listening involves the reception, decoding, and interpreting the aural stimuli. In simple terms, active listening is 'hearing for meaning'. Active listening does not mean the listener agrees with the speaker. On the contrary, the listener shows his understanding of what the speaker said. Active listening builds trust and avoids misunderstandings. It enables people to open up and to say more. The various stages of active listening are hearing, focusing on the message, comprehending and interpreting, analysing, responding, and, finally, remembering. Using correct body language, asking open questions (open questions lead to descriptive answers, while closed questions are answered with a short phrase), listening non-judgmentally, summarizing, reflecting, clarifying, and showing empathy are some of the means of listening actively.

Principles of effective communication (figure 2.2)

The following are the most important, basic principles of effective communication.

- It is important to set a goal at the beginning of the conversation.
- Effective communication is dependent not only on content (words), but also on context (body language, tone of voice, expression, etc.).
- When the speaker is talking, the recipient should listen actively (see above).
- Eliciting and evaluating feedback and determining if the recipients not only heard the speaker but also understood the meaning and intent will increase the effectiveness of communication.

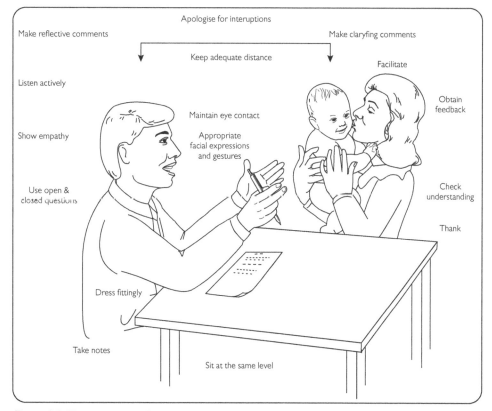

Figure 2.2 The components of good communication.

When providing feedback, use positive rather than negative feedback. Positive feedback is more readily and accurately sensed than negative feedback. The language used in feedback should be non-judgemental.

- It is important to find the right balance of the components of communication (setting goal, content, context, active listening, and feedback) and *any one aspect should not be overdone.*
- Always remember the five Cs of communication:
  - **Clarity** (being clear, distinct, and easily perceived)
  - **Completeness** (providing all the necessary or appropriate information)
  - **Conciseness** (giving information in few words)
  - **Concreteness** (being perceived by the senses; not abstract or imaginary)
  - **Correctness** (conforming to accepted standards).

Barriers to effective communication

- Patient- or doctor-related barriers:
  - Culture and personality differences between doctors and patients can interfere and change the meaning of the message conveyed.
  - Focusing on self: effective communication is about listening and focusing on the other person rather than self. Focusing on oneself might be either because of feeling of superiority ('I know more than you') or defensiveness ('If I let him ask anything, he will expose my ignorance').
  - Bias of perception: one may dismiss the speaker if he or she feels they are talking too fast or haltingly.
  - Environmental: bright lights and noise are potential distracters, which will affect the concentration of both the sender and the recipient and impede effective communication.
  - Language barriers.
- Doctor-related barriers:
  - Lack of good communication skills: many doctors do not understand the components of effective communication. Even among those who understand the basics, few practise and hone the skill.
  - Inadequate knowledge or training in context.
  - Lack of knowledge about the condition: this is not necessarily a barrier to effective communication, provided, the doctors are honest about the limit of their knowledge.
  - Fear of disagreeable response from patients: doctors expect an unfavourable response and present an incomplete or misleading picture to avoid this.
  - Stress, particularly from exams.
- Patient-related barriers:
  - Patients and their families may steer conversations away from difficult topics.
  - Shyness, confusion, and fear of death or disability.

Strategies to overcome barriers to effective communication

- General:
  - Plan the responses after the other person has finished and *not* while speaking.
  - Take brief notes, which will help to concentrate on what is being said.
- Speaking:
  - Encourage and allow others to talk.
  - One should not try to dominate the conversation.
  - Avoid finishing the sentences for others.

- ◆ Provide feedback at an optimum level and don't interrupt the other person endlessly.
- ◆ Answer a question with a statement and not with another question.
- Listening:
  - ◆ In general, one should spend more time listening than talking.
  - ◆ Avoid being preoccupied with your own thoughts while others are talking.

Effective communication—the practice

Patients want the doctor to 'listen' to them and give them enough time to discuss their problems. Unfortunately, in the communication station, the candidate is allowed only 9 minutes with the patient. The good candidate will be expected to prove competence in managing what is usually a difficult communication scenario in this limited time. Some of the commonly tested areas in the MRCPCH exam are given in table 2.2.

- Before entering the station:
  - ◆ Stay calm, read the scenario, and draw up a plan.
  - ◆ Avoid talking to others.
- Environment—the setting (figure 2.3):
  - ◆ Make sure you are dressed fittingly, as a neat, conservative appearance may be regarded as a sign of competence by the patient.
  - ◆ Ensure the room is comfortable with good lighting.
  - ◆ Set the examination room to promote and heighten the candidate–patient interaction. Arrange the furniture appropriately to encourage a sense of partnership between the child, parents, and the doctor. Never sit across the table. A preferred arrangement is to sit by adjacent sides of the table at the same level.
  - ◆ Remove distractions; switch off mobile phones and bleeps.
- Initial steps:
  - ◆ Introduce yourself: shake hands with the child and family members.
  - ◆ Clarify roles: explain why the meeting has been arranged.
  - ◆ Confidentiality: 'What ever we are discussing is confidential and between us only and will not be divulged to anyone else without your permission'.
  - ◆ Establish rapport.
  - ◆ Show empathy and respect.
  - ◆ Maintain eye contact throughout the meeting.
- Communication etiquette:
  - ◆ Address the child by their correct name and not just he or she. This shows your appreciation of the child's individuality and their presence.
  - ◆ Parents should be addressed in a formal style, for example as Mr and Mrs Smith, and not as mum or dad.
  - ◆ Ensure privacy for all sensitive communication. A patient is unlikely to reveal personal information if they think the person next door can hear what is being said.
  - ◆ If parents do not speak English fluently, ask for an interpreter.
  - ◆ Avoid making assumptions about the child and the family or sounding vague.
  - ◆ Avoid frequent interruptions and do not be dismissive of a patient's or parent's concerns.
  - ◆ Allow them to ask questions and answer them.
  - ◆ Do not argue with the parents, as their viewpoint can be valid and correct.
  - ◆ Show that you are listening actively, by:
    - ■ appropriate eye contact
    - ■ posture (for example, sitting forward facing the patient)

Table 2.2 Possible scenarios in the communication station

Category	Examples	Special comments
Giving information	Discussing a complex diagnosis, for example Guillain–Barré syndrome	Give accurate information Use simple, easy to understand language—avoid jargon Allow the family time to digest information—they can come back later for further information or discussion
	Ease distress and reassure, for example a mum worried about a thriving preschool child with chronic diarrhoea (you diagnosed toddler's diarrhoea), or a mum worried about MRSA outbreak in the NICU where her preterm baby is receiving care	Give accurate information Avoid the use of jargon Show empathy Acknowledge and respond to the child's and parents' emotions
	Explaining treatment, for example endocarditis prophylaxis	Give reasons and explain the likely benefits of therapy Possible side effects Ask whether they are likely to comply with the treatment
	Explaining a procedure, for example ventricular tap in a child with posthaemorrhagic hydrocephalus	Draw diagrams if possible Give parents time to react to information Allow questions
Breaking bad news	For example inform parents about a diagnosis of leukaemia, or a premature baby in special care with sudden worsening due to intraventricular haemorrhage	Build the bad news gradually Give accurate information about treatment options and outcome sensitively Avoid the use of jargon Show empathy Acknowledge and respond to the child's and parents' emotions Allow the patient time to react to information Leave room for hope Check understanding Allow time for questions Summarize information
	Accidental drug overdose in a health-care setting	Explain what has happened and how it happened Apologize sincerely for the error Give possible reasons for the accident What are the likely effects of this incident—how likely the child is to suffer harm What is being done to ensure that this will not happen in the future
Persuade	For example convince an adolescent with paracetamol poisoning who is refusing treatment	Give accurate information about treatment options and outcome sensitively Allow time to react to information Avoid the use of jargon Show empathy Acknowledge and respond to the child's emotions

Table 2.2 *Continued*

Category	Examples	Special comments
Responding to patient dissatisfaction	Dissatisfaction about treatment or some aspect of management, for example a delay in diagnosis or treatment	Understand why the patient or parent is angry Reflect on the patient's anger by putting it into words Acknowledge the patient's emotion Achieve a clear understanding of the patient's perspective Find common ground and steer the discussion away from the point of conflict Avoid confrontation Attempt to resolve the situation
Cross-cultural communication	Treatment compliance problems	Explore and clarify the problem Do not assume the patient cannot understand you Use an interpreter when necessary Work within the patient's framework of understanding Explore the patient's view within the norms of their culture Explore solutions within the patient's norms and terms of reference Involve other agencies as suggested
Discussing resuscitation status	Discussing a do not resuscitate order	Recognize this is a highly emotionally charged discussion Get the setting right Use appropriate language—no jargon Set the scene with an account of the patient's illness Explain the need for discussion on resuscitation Respond to family's emotions with empathy Discuss support and aftercare Offer an opportunity to ask questions and time for the family to come to terms with decisions Summarize

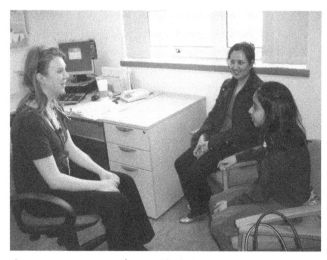

Figure 2.3 An environment to promote good communication.

- nodding your head
- encouraging the patient to 'go on'
- asking questions directly related to or following what has just been said.

  ♦ Facilitation: encouraging the patient to say what they want to say, for example saying 'please continue'.
  ♦ Clarification: make clear what you mean or what the patient means.
  ♦ Reflection: this is a remark expressed after careful consideration of the patient's words.
  ♦ Use of a pause or silence: there are moments when it may be necessary to pause or to remain silent to allow the patient to digest the information. Do not rush!
  ♦ Empathy: react to patient's state of mind and emotion. Give timely, kind words and a sympathetic look to an upset patient; for example you can say, 'I understand how you feel'.

- Information delivery:
  ♦ Before giving information, find out what the patient knows about their problem and its possible treatment.
  ♦ Identify and acknowledge the family's beliefs and worries.
  ♦ Use a combination of open and closed questions. Answers to questions depend on how the questions are asked.
  ♦ Patients and their families may be unwilling to express their real concerns, but may give verbal and non-verbal cues. You should pick up on these cues and explore them to get to the root cause of the problem.
  ♦ Outline what you will discuss and give the most important information first.
  ♦ Give information sensitively with empathy.
  ♦ Frame your answer in terms of what you know, while keeping the information specific and relevant.
  ♦ Use plain language with concise and clear wording. Avoid the use of medical terms. Do not assume the parents understand the meaning of some of the medical jargon. For example, any headache could be regarded as 'migraine' by parents.
  ♦ Allow moments of silence to reflect on the discussion.
  ♦ Take notes to focus and to show your seriousness in the conversation.
  ♦ Where suitable, use drawings to explain.
  ♦ Take into account the cultural views of the family.
  ♦ Deal with issues sensitively and try to alleviate anxiety.
  ♦ Check their understanding of information given.
  ♦ In defensive situations, for example if a parent asks a question that you may not know the answer to, be honest. Do not be afraid to say 'I don't know' or 'I am not really sure ... but I will find out or I will discuss this with the person who knows about the area of concern and get back to you'.
  ♦ Repeat or summarize your understanding at intervals.

- Behaviour:
  ♦ Stay quiet when the family is talking.
  ♦ Always be open and show it in your face and body language.
  ♦ Adopt a receptive posture.
  ♦ Have appropriate eye contact.
  ♦ Keep your arms open and don't cross them.
  ♦ Show appropriate facial expression and gestures.
  ♦ Do not keep thinking about what you are going to say next instead of listening.
  ♦ Observe and question judiciously as part of the listening process.

- Epilogue:
  - ◆ Towards the end of the interview, ask the child or the parent to summarize what has been discussed.
  - ◆ If you are running out of time, tell the parents that due to lack of time you will continue the discussion at a later time.
  - ◆ Summarize what you have said and what the patient has told you. It allows you to check the accuracy of information that has been exchanged.
  - ◆ Always close the conversation with a follow-up plan.
  - ◆ Enquire if they want to add anything.
  - ◆ End by thanking the child and the family.

Common scenarios: giving information

Failure to give information or a satisfactory explanation is the most common cause of dissatisfaction among patients. In most of the scenarios, the candidate will face a situation where they will be required to give information to the patient's family. Essential steps in giving information effectively are:

- understanding the information
- using plain language, which is easily understood by the recipient
- exploring the family's views on the information given
- when there is a conflict, trying to see the patient's view
- considering the cultural views of the family
- checking their understanding of information given
- responding to the questions and emotional reaction
- summarizing the main points of the discussion.

Common scenarios: breaking bad news

Breaking bad news is a vital skill for any MRCPCH exam candidate. Bad news is information that is perceived by patients and families to affect their future adversely. Breaking bad news is a challenging task which needs to be approached with skill and sensitivity. Keep an open mind on what is 'bad news'. Some patients are distressed by seemingly good news, while others experience some relief on hearing bad news. It is advisable to give bad news to both parents, along with anyone else who they feel might offer support. Ideally, information should be given in a suitable place free from interruptions (this is not relevant for exam purposes but is an important point to remember).

Key points of breaking bad news are as follows.

- Do it slowly or at a pace dictated by the patient or family.
- Show empathy: do not be afraid to lay a comforting hand on a shoulder.
- Clarify and remind the patient or family about confidentiality.
- Start with what the patient already knows (ICE,– Ideas (beliefs), Concerns, and Expectations).
- Find out what they want to know.
- Be attentive, listen, and give information sensitively.
- Elicit the patient's own resources for coping.
- Don't react defensively if the family becomes angry on hearing the news.
- Offer continuing support for the family, including counselling services.
- Instil realistic hope.
- Reassure the family that future meetings can be arranged if they feel it is necessary.
- Learn the cultural background of the family and how it influences their perceptions of disease and treatment. Be open-minded about cultural practices unfamiliar to you.

- Points to employ while communicating with children:
  - Adapt what you say to child's level of understanding. Relate to the child according to their developmental age. Learn what the child knows about illness and death.
  - Put yourself at the same level as the child while talking to them.
  - Learn the child's terminology for their concerns.
  - Engage the help of a parent or carer wherever possible.
  - Be honest. Do not lie or give false information or reassurance.
  - Repeat the information and check what the child has understood.
  - Play, drawings, and real-life examples can help the child to understand disability and loss.
  - Attend to the needs and concerns of parents and siblings, who are sometimes more distressed than the child.
  - Accept that bad temper and temper tantrums are normal reactions.
  - Allow time for questions and concerns.
- Points to avoid while communicating with children:
  - Rely too much on bribery or small gifts.
  - Make promises you cannot keep, for example 'this won't hurt'.
  - Use complex language, which the child will not understand.
  - Patronize—particularly true with adolescents!
- At the end of the session, check the parents' and the child's understanding:
  - Review and prioritize the problems
  - Work out an agreed management plan and follow-up.
  - Give time to ask questions: 'Is there anything you wish to ask me?'
  - Thank the family for their time.

Videos

Video 2.1 In this station Dr Helen Price talks to a young mother whose baby has been found to have an unexplained fracture of the arm. She communicates effectively by introducing herself, clarifying her role, showing appropriate empathy, and avoiding the use of medical jargon. She maintains good eye contact and demonstrates appropriate body language. Dr Price listens to the mother and answers her questions. Finally, she summarizes all the key points at the end of the discussion.

Video 2.2 In this video, Dr King examines a candidate who is breaking bad news to a mum whose infant was in a special care baby unit. You will notice that the candidate does show empathy and makes an effort to explain the underlying problem but she also uses a lot of medical jargon, which is pointed out both by the mum and the examiner. At the end, Dr King gives her feedback on her performance.

Chapter 3 **Focused history taking**

Focused history taking is a vital part of the MRCPCH clinical exam; candidates are expected to grasp the key issues and formulate an effective management plan. This station requires candidates to be efficient, purposeful, and well-directed in their approach. The candidate is expected to obtain and present the key facts in the history and suggest an appropriate management plan. The examiner sits in the room as an observer while the candidate takes the history. This gives the examiner ample opportunity to assess the candidate's communication skills, general approach, and knowledge of the condition. Only 13 minutes are allowed with the patient in the presence of the examiner. In the subsequent 9 minutes, the candidate will present and discuss the history. *Problem-oriented history and management is the most effective way of approaching this station.*

The objectives of obtaining a focused paediatric history are:

- to establish and maintain rapport with the child and parents
- to obtain an overview of the child's previous and current health issues
- to establish the psychological, family, and social context of a child's illness
- to reach a correct diagnosis (or form a differential diagnosis)
- to plan an appropriate management strategy.

Although the principles of history taking in children are similar to those used for adults, there are important differences in the scheme and the details. The paediatric case history is potentially more difficult to elicit and is influenced by the age of the child. For each age group, you will have to adapt your style. The primary historian may be the child or another person, usually the parent. The consultation itself is triadic, involving the child, their family (or caregiver), and the doctor. *Always keep in mind the principles of communication (discussed in chapter 2) and use an empathic approach while taking the history.*

Although in most cases the parents give the history, the child must also be encouraged to speak. In young children who have limited speech, you must take the history through the parents or the carers. In teenagers, there is a difficult line to tread between giving the child complete autonomy and allowing the parent to be the main historian. The better approach would be to allow both parties to contribute equally. In some cases this can be very challenging, as there may be conflicting accounts. In such instances, as the patient is the child and not the parent, focus your attention on the child's story whist engaging the parents. In general, children older than 4 years understand what is being said and should be allowed to contribute to the history. Often, teenagers may wish to give the history themselves without the parent. If the child or family is not well versed in English, seek an interpreter.

At the outset, it is essential to establish rapport with the child and the parents. As emphasized in chapter 2, it is important to listen actively to the parents and the child. Encourage the child to speak. Do not be dismissive of the child's or parent's concerns. Allow them to ask questions and answer them as truthfully and honestly as possible. The dictum 'the parents are always right, unless proved otherwise' is invariably true.

Time management is crucial for success in this station. Patients always want a doctor to *listen* to them and give them enough time. Given the limited available time, keep the history relevant and *focused*. Avoid asking the diagnosis at the start, as the history will give the cues to the possible diagnosis. Remember, just getting the correct diagnosis does not guarantee success. It is the principles used to get there that the examiner is looking for. Key competence skills required during focused history taking are given in table 3.1.

Principles of focused history taking

The preparation

The following section will guide and help you prepare for focused history taking in a systematic manner. Practise history taking and communication with a colleague using some of the common scenarios

Table 3.1 Key competence skills required in history taking

Competence skill	Standard
Understand the process and appreciate the difference in obtaining a paediatric medical history in comparison to an adult	Ability to obtain a focused paediatric history in a limited time Demonstrate this skill in the triadic consultation with the child, their family, and the doctor
Understand how the age of the child has an impact on medical history	Ability to engage the child and value their contribution
Demonstrate competence in the use of open-ended and closed questions	Ability to employ both open and closed question while taking a paediatric history Use proper wording of open-ended and directed questions
Understand the importance of various elements of history in a paediatric patient	Demonstrate ability for focused history taking when time is limited and avoid obtaining superfluous information not relevant to the main problems Obtain history on various aspects including perinatal history, birth history, development, immunization, family and social history
Demonstrate competence in summarizing and presenting to the examiner logically information gathered in history taking	Ability to synthesize the information gathered into a coherent, logical history Ability to think through the information gathered and explain any conflicts identified
Create an appropriate list of differential diagnosis, investigations, and management plan	Ability to form differential diagnosis and an appropriate management plan including relevant investigations
Understand the role of the multidisciplinary team in managing complex chronic conditions	Identify the relevant key members of the multidisciplinary team who may be required for the management of children with complex problems

listed in table 3.2. You can also ask your registrars and consultants to watch you take histories in routine clinical practice and get some useful feedback. There is only one way to master this station—practise taking and presenting the history again and again.

In the exam, *put yourself in the place of the child or the parent before taking a history*. This will give you some insight into their problems. You should adopt a systematic approach to taking a history and come up with a list of problems, even if the diagnosis is known. While taking a history, try to identify the features that support your diagnosis.

Two minutes before entering the station

Before entering the station, read the scenario carefully and identify the objectives clearly. Decide the outline and the point of origin of the interview. Quickly note down important points that you should address. As already mentioned, remember the child's name, age, and sex, as well as the caregiver's name, before you start talking. In the exam, you will have 13 minutes to get the history. Use 9 minutes to take the history and 4 minutes to complete, summarize, and recheck the history.

Environment—the setting

- Make sure you are dressed fittingly for the exam. Remember, good conservative dressing may be positively regarded by the patient as a sign of competence.
- Ensure the room is comfortable with good lighting.
- Set the exam room to promote and facilitate candidate–patient interaction. Arrange the furniture appropriately to encourage a sense of partnership between the child, parents, and the doctor.

Table 3.2 Possible cases in a focused history station

Disease	Important associated problems
Genetic conditions	
Trisomy 21 (Down's syndrome)	Cardiac defects, learning difficulties, hypothyroidism, speech and language problems
Turner's syndrome (XO)	Cardiac defects, learning difficulties, growth problems
Cri-du-chat syndrome	Cardiac defects, learning difficulties, growth problems
Noonan's syndrome	Cardiac defects, growth problems
Williams' syndrome	Cardiac defects such as supravalvular aortic stenosis, pulmonary stenosis, learning difficulties
22q11 Deletion syndromes (di George, velocardiofacial syndrome)	Cardiac defects, learning difficulties, endocrine problems
Neurofibromatosis type 1	Multiple system involvement (cardiac, skeletal, renal), psychological
Tuberous sclerosis	Epilepsy, learning difficulties
Marfan's syndrome	Growth issues, cardiac complications, psychological
Friedreich's ataxia	Neurological (ataxia), cardiac problems, genetics
Inflammatory conditions	
Inflammatory bowel disease (Crohn's disease or ulcerative colitis)	Chronic abdominal pain, altered bowel habits, poor growth, anaemia
Metabolic conditions	
Diabetes mellitus (type 1)	Usually type 1, poorly controlled, non-compliant teenager
Cystic fibrosis	Growth failure, recurrent respiratory tract infections, diabetes
Birth trauma and neonatal problems	
Cerebral palsy	Different types of cerebral palsy, movement disorder, speech and language problems, learning difficulties
Premature infant with complications	Developmental delay, speech and language problems, visual, learning difficulties, attention deficit hyperactive disorder
Biliary atresia	Previous surgery such as Kasai procedure or liver transplant, medications: immunosuppressives
Miscellaneous	
Nephrotic syndrome	Recurrent relapses, immunosuppressive use, complications of long-term steroid use
Coeliac disease	Gluten sensitivity, growth failure, special diet

Never sit across the table. A preferred sitting arrangement is to sit by adjacent sides of the table at the same level.
- Remove distractions—switch off mobile phones.

General principles
- Introduce yourself and shake hands with the patient and family members.
- Clarify the objective—explain why the meeting has been arranged.

- Establish a rapport—it may be appropriate to use a toy to establish rapport with a preschool child. Starting the conversation on a lighter note, such as talking about the weather or a current subject of interest, will usually put the family at ease.
- Show empathy and respect.
- Address the patient by their correct name and not just 'he' or 'she'. Parents may be addressed in a formal style as Mr and Mrs Smith, not as 'mum' or 'dad'.
- If parents do not speak English, get an interpreter.
- Maintain eye contact throughout the meeting.
- Start with open questions followed by closed questions.
- Keep a logical flow of content.
- Note down important points only and give the child undivided attention. Avoid writing too much and losing eye contact.
- Speak clearly in plain language without the use of medical jargon. For example it is better to avoid terms such as pneumonia, instead say chest infection. If you use a medical term, explain what you mean and use these sparingly.
- Find out how the family and the child feel about the problem and focus on the patient's perspective of the illness.
- Keep in mind the **communication etiquette** discussed in chapter 2 and follow this during history taking. Remember, the examiner is evaluating both your history taking and communication skills.
- In the final 4 minutes:
  - Check the list of the objectives which you prepared before the interview and complete any missed points.
  - Ask the child and or parents 'What is most worrying for you?'
  - Ask them 'Is there anything important I didn't ask?'
  - Summarize and clarify the history making sure all important aspects have been covered.
- Thank them for coming to see you before they leave the room.

Outline of the paediatric history

Gather information under the following headings:

- identifying data such as names and addresses
- chief complaint and history of presenting illness
- review of other systems—keep it concise in a paediatric case history; this is more helpful with older children and teenagers
- past history:
  - medical
  - current medications
  - periconception
  - antenatal
  - perinatal, especially for a young child
  - neonatal
- immunization history
- developmental history
- family history
- social history.

Identifying data

- full name and nickname
- sex
- date of birth and age
- full name of each parent
- address and contact details of the child and each parent
- phone numbers of each parent.

Chief complaint

The chief complaint is a brief description of why the child presented for medical care. Depending on the child's age, it should be recorded in the parent's or child's own words. Where there are multiple symptoms, list them depending on their relevance, their relationships, and the duration of each symptom.

History of the presenting illness

In the history of the presenting illness, the details of the chief complaint should be expanded. Establish the date of onset when appropriate. Obtain a concise chronological account of the illness, with a full description of symptoms (suitable positive history) and relevant negatives from the onset to the present time. Try to disentangle the facts instead of accepting the parents' interpretation. Allow them to tell the history in their own way and later ask specific questions to fill in the necessary details. The effect of medication on the chief symptom and any investigations, tests, or radiological studies that have been done so far should also be noted.

Questions to ask about the current illness include:

- When and how did it start?
- Was the child well before symptoms started?
- How did it develop?
- What aggravates or relieves the symptoms?
- What is the outline of the course of the symptom?
- Have there been any earlier episodes of a similar illness?
- Are there any other members of the family or friends with similar symptoms?
- How has the illness affected the family?
- How is the symptom affecting the child's life (such as lost nursery or schooldays)?

Systems review

After the history of the presenting complaint, it may be necessary to review briefly other systems to check for their involvement. This may not be always necessary and it should be kept concise. Ask questions relevant to the diagnostic hypotheses and use a systematic approach to evaluate the symptoms.

- general: fever, recent weight change, activity level, ability to keep up with peers
- head: injuries, headache
- eyes: discharge, redness, puffiness, vision-related problems
- ears: difficulty in hearing, discharge, tinnitus, vertigo
- nose: congestion, epistaxis
- mouth: sore throat, swallowing difficulty, dental problems
- respiratory: breathlessness, cough, wheeze, hoarseness, haemoptysis, chest pain
- cardiovascular: breathlessness, palpitation, syncope, oedema, exercise tolerance

- gastrointestinal: vomiting, abdominal pain, frequency of bowel movements, jaundice
- urinary: dysuria, frequency, urgency, nocturia, haematuria, menarche
- neurological: altered consciousness, weakness, numbness, fainting, incoordination, tremors, seizures
- musculoskeletal: deformities, pain, swelling, warmth, muscle cramps, gait changes
- skin: rashes, itching
- allergy: urticaria, hay fever, asthma, eczema
- sexual history: this should be asked sensitively, with questions such as 'Some youngsters of your age are sexually active. How about you?', and may be best asked in parents' absence. Other points include onset and regularity of menarche in females, dysmenorrhoea, and onset of pubertal changes in boys.

Past history

- Medical: obtain the history about the child's significant past medical problems. Areas that should be covered include:
  - reasons for continuing care
  - teams providing the continuing care
  - past hospitalizations
  - medications
  - surgeries
  - recent travel abroad or visitors from foreign countries.
- Current medications: it is worth remembering that the parent's memory of medication may not be accurate; some parents do not consider over the counter drugs to be medication. Look at the prescriptions and GP letters for corroboration, which also serve as useful sources of additional information. It is important to enquire about adverse drug reactions, which often are perceived inappropriately as allergies.
  - prescribed medication: dose, route, duration
  - over the counter medication
  - complementary or homeopathic medicine
  - adverse reactions and allergies.
- Periconception period: the relative importance of the following items depends on the age of the child and the reason for the visit. The younger the child, the more detailed the history of pregnancy should be. Important questions to ask are:
  - Was there any maternal illness around time of conception?
  - Was the child conceived naturally or by assisted reproduction?
  - If relevant, establish whether the child was adopted or in foster care, with due sensitivity to the child's awareness of the facts.
- Antenatal history: any factors relevant to maternal and fetal well-being should be recorded:
  - mother's age at delivery
  - previous pregnancies and their outcome, including history of pregnancy loss (spontaneous or induced)
  - maternal medical history (e.g. antenatal infections)
  - obstetric complications (diabetes, pregnancy-induced hypertension, oligohydramnios, polyhydramnios, rhesus incompatibility, antepartum haemorrhage)
  - maternal exposure to prescribed medications or recreational substance at the time of conception and throughout the pregnancy
  - level of antenatal care
  - investigations (first trimester screening, amniocentesis, radiology)

- maternal smoking and alcohol intake: how many cigarettes and how much alcohol per day
- fetal growth and well-being.
- Perinatal (birth) history: factors relevant to the child's health should be identified.
  - gestation
  - duration of labour
  - type of delivery (normal vaginal, forceps, vacuum extraction, Caesarean section, spontaneous or induced)
  - place of delivery (hospital, birthing centre, home) and who attended the delivery (doctor, nurse, midwife)
  - interventions in the delivery room, if any
  - birth weight
  - congenital malformations.
- Neonatal history: relevant questions to ask about the neonatal period include:
  - length of stay in the hospital after birth
  - neonatal illnesses (feeding problems, infections, hypoglycaemia, hypothermia, anaemia, convulsions, respiratory distress, or jaundice)
  - need for special care or intensive care
  - use of oxygen or respiratory support
  - Guthrie test, normally recorded in the Red Book.

Immunization history

The history should contain the list of the immunizations the child has received and reactions, if any. Avoid unhelpful statements such as 'immunizations are up-to-date'. Be specific about the vaccines the child has received and highlight the ones that have been missed. It is useful to glance quickly through the personal health record (or Red Book) to get a full picture of immunizations and early development.

Developmental history

Developmental history is important in the younger child. In the older child, performance at school should be included besides the developmental history. It may be useful to compare the child's progress and milestones with that of siblings and peers. For details, refer to chapter 11.

- ages of attainment of major milestones in all major streams of development—gross motor, language, fine motor–adaptive (including cognitive and fine motor), and personal–social; current developmental abilities—smiling, rolling, sitting alone, crawling, walking, running, first word, toilet training, riding tricycle, etc.
- attendance at day care, preschool, or school
  - When did the child start school?
  - How well is the child doing, are there any concerns?
  - Any additional support at school?
  - specific questions about progress in individuals subjects such as reading, spelling and mathematics
  - interaction with peers
- behaviour:
  - normal sleep–wake cycle, alertness and activity
  - issues such as enuresis, temper tantrums, thumb sucking, head-banging, night terrors
- emotional history—specific questions may be asked about:
  - hobbies and interests
  - emotionally disturbing life events, where appropriate, such as family break-up

- feeding history:
  - initial feeding—breast or bottle (How often? How much? Why and any supplements)?
  - weaning—introduction of solids (including quality and quantity of solids, meal frequency, adverse reactions to foods)
  - nutritional supplementation
  - current intake
    - fluid (including milk, juice, water, and beverages)
    - food (How many meals does your child eat? Favourite foods?).

Family history

Gathering a complete and accurate family history is important, particularly in genetic diseases. Create a family tree that includes the last two generations. Ask specific questions about the family that are related to the child's chief complaint. For example if the child has rectal bleeding, ask for history of inflammatory bowel disease. In addition, ask specifically about:

- the age of the parents and the siblings
- history of consanguinity and ethnic background
- health of the father, mother, siblings, and grandparents
- whether any other member of the family has the same condition
- in case of genetic conditions in the family, ask for the age of onset
- any deaths, ages at death, and causes of death
- if the child is adopted, ask the adoptive parents about any known family history.

Social history

This is separate from family history but is allied to it. It is the summary of lifestyle practices, which may have a direct or indirect effect on a person's health and is a sensitive part of the history. Take care not to offend when enquiring about the family by making assumptions about who may be present or 'involved'. Be prepared to allow information to come out gradually. Ask about the following:

- person-related:
  - parent's occupation/ employment
  - who provides childcare if both parents are working?
  - major life events—have there been any recent deaths, accidents, or divorce?
  - substance abuse—problems with alcohol or drugs
  - marital stability—do parents live together?
  - who has parental responsibility?
- environment-related:
  - home environment
  - how many bedrooms?
  - how many occupants?
  - housing benefits
  - any modification to the home in cases of disability
  - does anyone in the family smoke?
  - any pets
- economics-related:
  - finances, including aid—is the family on income support?
  - support systems—relatives and friends
  - recreational history—play, respite care.

Special case: history from a teenager

- Points to employ
  - ◆ Gain the patient's confidence.
  - ◆ Make sure ground rules and objectives are clear right from the start.
  - ◆ Start the interview with one of the parents initially. Later, talk to the teenager alone, particularly regarding sensitive issues, as some may be unwilling to communicate in the presence of a parent. Give assurance that confidentiality and privacy are guaranteed.
  - ◆ Make them understand why you need to ask certain questions.
  - ◆ Let them tell their problem in their own words.
  - ◆ Show interest in what the teenager and not the parent has to say. Encourage by saying 'I want to hear what you think'.
  - ◆ Non-verbal cues are important in a teenager: looks, gestures, signs, and facial expressions. Expressions of approval for positive attributes and suitably placed expressions of empathy will go a long way in making teenagers comfortable. A sense of humour will help ease tension.
  - ◆ Sensitive topics such as substance abuse, sexuality, anxiety, depression, eating disorders, and family dysfunction must be handled carefully and left for the latter half of the interview when rapport is established.
  - ◆ Ask about social habits—smoking, alcohol, hobbies, etc.
  - ◆ Ask about sexual history when relevant. Keep in mind the possibility of pregnancy!
- Points to avoid
  - ◆ Do not start with the sensitive issues.
  - ◆ Do not be heavy handed with a difficult teenager.

Summarize information

At the end of session, check the parent's and the child's understanding.

- Review and rank the problems identified.
- Give the child and parents time to ask questions 'Is there anything you wish to ask me?'
- Work out an agreed management plan and follow up.
- Thank the family for their time.

Discussion with the examiner

- Give a concise presentation—try presenting from memory, only using written notes as a guide!
- Focus on the main points.
- Explore the impact of the illness on the child and the family.
- Offer a differential diagnosis—keep it short and concise and include only conditions that could explain all the child's symptoms and signs.
- Have a clear management plan.
- For investigations, always start with the least expensive, least painful, least invasive tests that offer the greatest likelihood of confirming the diagnosis.

Video

Video 3.1 In this station on focused history taking, Dr Helen Price obtains a good history by introducing herself, clarifying her role, and asking both open-ended and closed questions. She maintains good eye contact and has appropriate body language. Dr Price does not interrupt the history taking. She engages both the child and the mother in the conversation. To conclude, she summarizes and formulates an appropriate management plan.

Chapter 4 The principles of physical examination

Examination of the child combines science with art; developing competence in paediatric examination requires both knowledge of the correct technique and hours of hard work and practise. Lack of either will make the examination technique incomplete or inadequate. Perhaps the greatest difficulty an inexperienced doctor faces is to gain the confidence and trust of the child and their carers, while creating an impression of grounded self-confidence.

In the examination, one should carry oneself well. This means you should be a good listener, be interested, cheerful, respectful, warm, caring, friendly, empathic, competent, and diplomatic. It is imperative to listen actively to the child and their carers and be as natural as possible—just as you would be with your friend's child or indeed your own.

The examination begins the moment you enter the room. It is essential to understand that the general approach to the physical examination of the child will be different from that of an adult and will vary according to the age of the child. As the child's cooperation cannot be guarantied, you should remember that it is impossible always to use a set protocol while examining the child. We have listed the essential steps of examination in a particular order so that all areas are covered, but *the candidate needs to adapt the examination sequence according to the needs of the child and the situation.* As a general rule, anything that will inevitably be uncomfortable or unpleasant for the child (e.g. otoscopy or rectal examination) should be the 'last act' of the examination.

A common mistake made by nervous candidates is to talk too fast; this is a trait that will always be more exaggerated under the stress of the exam. Pausing at the end of each sentence is an effective way of slowing down. Ensuring that each word is pronounced completely will also lessen the pace of your speech. Talking slowly and clearly with a smile on your face will help to hide nervousness.

General approach

In this book and the accompanying videos, examinations are performed in a systematic manner. These steps provide a useful framework. Although there can be some flexibility, following the steps listed here will improve your technique. Make sure you observe the following:

- infection control
- introduction, patient identification, and consent
- establishing rapport with the child and parents
- ensuring privacy of the patient
- positioning the patient correctly
- making a visual survey—head to toe examination
- system examination, which should include:
  - inspection
  - palpation
  - percussion
  - auscultation
- examination of other relevant systems.

The following paragraphs describe in detail some of the steps that will help you to conduct the examination professionally. These need to be repeated in every case, irrespective of the case scenario.

Infection control

- *On entering the examination room, show strict adherence to infection control by washing your hands or using alcohol rub.*
- If you are wearing a long-sleeved shirt, roll it up above the elbow to be 'bare below the elbows'.

Introduction, patient identification, and consent

Introduce yourself *both* to the parents and the child in a warm friendly manner. A handshake may be suitable for an older child. Kneel down or sit in a low chair to get down to the level of the child. Use toys to help you gain the cooperation of infants and toddlers. Give your name and explain the purpose of your visit.

The following is an example of an introduction.

- 'Hello, I am Dr X.'
- 'Thank you for letting me examine your child.' (Avoid asking a question such as 'Can I examine you? If the child says 'no', you are in real trouble!)
- *Ask the name and age of the child, if not already told by the examiner.*
- *Always address the child by their correct name.*

Establishing rapport with the child and parents

- Do not jump to the examination straight away. Be calm and do not rush.
- Try to start a conversation with the child. A short time spent establishing rapport will help in gaining the child's confidence and cooperation. You may do this by appreciating the child's dress, their toys, or their gadgets if they are older. With teenagers, it might be more useful to talk about their hobbies or their sport idols.
- Listen carefully to the 'examiner's opening statement'. For example if you are examining an 8-year-old child and the examiner talks about 'recurrent aspiration as an infant', this might be a clue as to why the child has subsequently developed bronchiectasis, the signs of which you would then be expected to elicit.

Factors important for establishing rapport include:

- Address the child by name.
- Keep appropriate eye contact with the child.
- Listen attentively to anything the child says and engage in conversation. However, be careful that you do not significantly cut short the time available for your examination and if necessary interject with 'I am sorry to stop our discussion about X, but can you tell me a little bit more about Y'.)
- Give the child your undivided attention.

Ensure privacy

- Make sure to draw the curtains and get the child's permission before undressing them. Always ask the parent to help in undressing an older child (when required). For toddlers and preschool children, ask the parent to undress them, as it is less threatening to the child.
- Do not take even the youngest child for granted. We have come across 3 year olds who have suggested pulling the curtains before they remove their shirt!
- Avoid undressing a child yourself, especially children of secondary school age.
- Avoid undressing older girls, particularly teenagers. Wherever possible request the help of the parent.
- As a general rule, always have a chaperone when examining a child, irrespective of their age or sex.

Positioning the patient

This depends on the system being examined and will be discussed in more detail in subsequent chapters. In general, it is better to start the visual examination in whatever position the child is, before moving them to the position that is likely to yield most of the clinical findings. It is preferable to examine preschool children on their carer's lap—they will feel much more relaxed.

Basic methods of examination

A systematic approach to the examination will enable the candidate to identify any abnormal physical finding and to assess its significance.

Inspection

Inspection involves looking for physical signs by simple visual observation. One must do this first before anything else. If you do not observe the child at the start before diving in with your hands, you may miss something important and you may even end up making the wrong diagnosis. *This seemingly 'easy' skill is the most difficult one to learn, yet it could yield the maximum number of physical signs.* Often, candidates do not give enough importance to this skill, as it appears as though 'nothing is being done'. Inspection should start from the first moment of contact with the patient and can be considered **general** or **local.**

1. General inspection is the preliminary act of studying the body as a whole. Looking at the child as a whole gives the composite picture. The points to note are activity, build, growth, behaviour, speech, appearance of illness, dysmorphism, and many more, which are discussed in detail in the relevant chapters.
2. Local inspection focuses on a single region. The findings to be noted vary with the system and are discussed in the relevant chapters.

Palpation

Use the tip of the fingers for palpation, as they are the most sensitive areas for tactile discrimination. Palpation is done in two stages: **light** palpation and **deep** palpation. Always ask the child if any area is painful before continuing with the examination. While palpating, look for the texture and temperature of the skin. Describe in detail the size, shape, consistency, tenderness, mobility, and pulsation (expansile or transmitted) of any underlying organ or mass.

Percussion

There are two types of percussion: **direct**, where the object is percussed with the fingers, and **indirect**, in which percussion is performed over the pleximeter finger which is placed firmly on the body. There are four types of percussion sounds: resonant, hyper-resonant, dull, and stony dull. A dull sound suggests the presence of a solid mass under the surface. A resonant sound points to underlying air-containing structures.

Auscultation

Auscultation for the internal sounds of the body is relevant when examining the cardiovascular, respiratory, and abdominal systems or where a mass has been identified.

The relative importance of each of these techniques will depend on the system being examined but an attempt should be made to use them all to ensure that the physical examination has been completed.

Chapter 5 **Examination of the cardiovascular system**

All candidates taking the MRCPCH clinical examination will be expected to show competency in carrying out the cardiovascular examination. It is important to listen carefully to the examiner's instructions and follow them. You may be asked only to auscultate the heart. If the examiner gives such an instruction, simply follow it!

Important—before you proceed

You are advised to buy a good paediatric stethoscope, as it can reduce the difficulty in identifying cardiac sounds. The diaphragm of the stethoscope is designed to amplify high-pitched sounds; the bell does not amplify sound but transmits low-pitched sounds better than the diaphragm. The bell should be placed lightly against the skin, while the diaphragm should be placed firmly on the skin for ideal sound amplification and transmission. It is possible to make the bell act like a diaphragm by placing it firmly against the skin.

Examination of the cardiovascular system is best done in correlation with the available medical history, as this often gives major clues. It is helpful to have a systematic approach to presenting the findings, which of course should be practised thoroughly. *However, the examination itself can be performed in a different sequence depending on the age of the child and their degree of cooperation.*

Key competence skills required in the cardiovascular examination are given in table 5.1. Cardiovascular cases commonly encountered in the MRCPCH Clinical Exam are listed in table 5.2.

General approach

These steps are repeated in every system to reiterate their importance and to help you recollect the initial approach for any clinical exam. Also, refer to chapter 4.

Table 5.1 Key competence skills required in cardiovascular examination

Competence skill	Standard
Knowledge of descriptive terms of the cardiovascular system	Ability to use correct terminology for findings of cardiovascular system examination
Understanding the importance of correct positioning of the patient	Show ability to position the child correctly with optimal exposure of the chest
Knowledge and clear understanding of how to carry out a complete cardiovascular examination	Demonstrate a systematic approach to cardiovascular examination, which includes inspection, palpation, percussion, and auscultation
	Demonstrate the ability to recognize associated abnormalities such as clubbing of fingers or splinter haemorrhages
	Demonstrate the ability to identify heart sounds, splitting of heart sounds, added sounds, and murmurs (with relevant grading)
	Ability to look for clinical evidence of heart failure such crackles in lung bases, hepatomegaly, and to look for dependent oedema (sacral or ankle)
Understanding that some congenital syndromes may have associated characteristic cardiac anomalies	Demonstrate ability to look for evidence of dysmorphology of syndromes such as Down's syndrome, Turner's syndrome, Williams' syndrome, Marfan's syndrome
Summarize findings, offer a differential diagnosis, and discuss a management plan	Demonstrate the ability to coherently present findings and offer a differential diagnosis
	Give possible explanations for any inconsistencies identified
	Demonstrate the ability to offer an appropriate management plan

Table 5.2 Cardiovascular conditions that may be seen in the MRCPCH clinical exam

Primary cause	Disease	Associated heart defects
Congenital	Trisomy 21 (Down's syndrome)	AVSD, VSD, ASD
	Trisomy 18 (Edward's syndrome)	VSD
	Turners syndrome (XO)	CoA, AS
	Cri-du-chat (deletion of short arm of chromosome 5)	VSD
	Noonan's syndrome	PS (valve), hypertrophic cardiomyopathy
	Williams' syndrome	AS (supravalvar), pulmonary artery branch stenosis
	22q11 deletion (di George) syndrome	Interrupted aortic arch, truncus arteriosus, TOF
	Holt–Oram syndrome	ASD, VSD
	Congenital rubella syndrome	PDA, VSD
	Infant of diabetic mother	Septal hypertrophy, transposition of great arteries, VSD
	Maternal systemic lupus erythematosus–fetal lupus	Congenital heart block
	Fetal alcohol syndrome	ASD, VSD
	Fetal valproate syndrome	AS, PS, CoA, TOF
Metabolic conditions	Pompe's disease (type 2 glycogen storage disease)	Cardiomyopathy
	Familial hypercholesterolaemia	Tendon xanthomata, corneal arcus before puberty
	Mucopolysaccharidosis	Regurgitation or stenosis of valves
Infective conditions	Rheumatic fever	MS, MR, AS, AR, myocarditis, pericarditis
	Infective endocarditis	AR, MR
Connective tissue disorders	Marfan's syndrome	AR, mitral valve prolapse
	Ehlers–Danlos syndrome	MR, AR, aortic dissection
Degenerative disorders	Friedreich's ataxia	Cardiomyopathy in an older child with abnormal gait

AVSD, atrioventricular septal defect; VSD, ventricular septal defect; ASD, atrial septal defect; AS, aortic stenosis; PS, pulmonary stenosis; MS, mitral stenosis; MR, mitral regurgitation; AR, aortic regurgitation; TOF, tetralogy of Fallot; CoA, coarctation of the aorta; PDA, patent ductus arteriosus.

- *On entering the examination room, demonstrate strict adherence to infection control measures by washing your hands or using alcohol rub.*
- Introduce yourself *both* to the parents and the child.
- Talk slowly and clearly with a smile on your face.
- Establish rapport with the child and parents.
- Undress the child to the waist to allow proper examination. Expose adequately while ensuring their privacy.
- Positioning: it is easier to examine older children while they sit on the edge of the bed, or on a chair when they are not acutely ill. It is preferable to examine younger children on their parent's lap rather than on a couch away from the parents. Removing a toddler or an infant from his or her parents will probably yield a screaming child, which decreases the chances of correctly identifying the clinical signs.

Visual survey—head to toe examination

The aim of the visual survey is to 'capture' every available clue, which may help in arriving at the correct diagnosis.

- Look and try to estimate the approximate age of the child.
- Always think whether the findings combine to form a recognizable clinical syndrome. Common syndromes with cardiac involvement include Down's syndrome, Turner's syndrome, Williams' syndrome, Noonan's syndrome, Marfan's syndrome and 22q11 deletion syndrome (di George syndrome).
- Look and comment on the following:
  - state of wakefulness
  - general well-being—well or ill
  - nutrition and growth—*comment that you would like to plot the child's height and weight on a growth chart*
  - resting position
  - interest in the surroundings
  - size of the child
  - pink or pale in air or cyanosed
  - degree of respiratory distress
  - noise—grunting, wheeze, cough
  - environment (equipment)—oxygen mask, nasal cannula, intravenous catheter, pulse oximetry, feeding tube, gastrostomy
  - head:
    - size: microcephaly/ macrocephaly
    - shape: dolichocephaly (commonly seen in ex-preterm infants)
  - face: certain syndromes have characteristic dysmorphic features and an association with heart conditions (be careful about using the term 'dysmorphic' features, as parents may get upset): malar flush (rare in children) is seen in mitral stenosis; in conjunctiva (palpebral and bulbar), look for pallor and jaundice
  - mouth: look for the presence of teeth (age appropriate) and dental caries, which may be a source of infective endocarditis in congenital heart disease
  - tongue: colour (pallor, cyanosis, jaundice); distinguish between central cyanosis (bluish extremities and mucous membranes) and peripheral cyanosis (bluish extremities only)
  - hands: pallor, palmar crease, tuberous and tendon xanthomata (familial hypercholesterolaemia)
  - fingers: number (preaxial or postaxial accessory digits), clubbing, cyanosis, Osler's nodes (tender swellings at fingertips) in infective endocarditis
  - nails: splinter (linear) haemorrhages in infective endocarditis
  - difference in colour between the limbs.

General tactile examination

Pulse (figure 5.1)

- Pulse rate (count for 15 seconds and multiply by four; however, tell the examiner that, ideally, you would like to count for 1 minute).
- The clinically relevant pulses that should be palpated in a child are:
  - radial
  - brachial

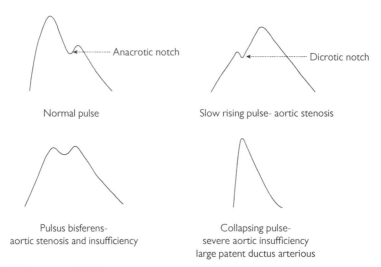

Figure 5.1 Different types of pulses.

- ◆ carotid (never palpate both carotids simultaneously as this can induce syncope)
- ◆ femoral (*do not forget to feel for femoral pulses*)
- ◆ dorsalis pedis (important if any scars are present in the groin).
- • Palpate the brachial pulse in an infant or toddler and radial pulse in older children.
- • Check both the right and left radial pulse, especially if there a history of dysphagia or airway obstruction or lateral thoracotomy scars (figure 5.2).
- • Comment on:
  - ◆ rate:
    - ▪ tachycardia—pulse rate above 100 beats per minute in children older than 3 years
    - ▪ bradycardia—pulse rate of less than 50 beats per minute is found in complete heart block or in children on drugs such as beta blockers or digoxin (rare in children)

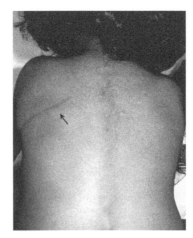

Figure 5.2 Left lateral thoracotomy scar.

- unequal or absent pulses with appropriate scars may be suggestive of specific surgery and may help with your diagnosis, e.g. Absent left radial pulse in post Blalock–Taussig shunt, repaired coarctation of the aorta, cervical rib;
  - feel both the radial and femoral pulses simultaneously and determine if there is any radiofemoral delay, a finding seen in coarctation of aorta
- rhythm:
  - **regularly irregular**—pulsus bigeminus, coupled extrasystoles, Wenckebach phenomenon (common in sleep, rare when awake)
  - **irregularly irregular**—multiple extrasystoles; ventricular extrasystoles are common in normal children and often disappear with exercise; atrial fibrillation causes an irregularly irregular pulse but is very rare in children
- volume:
  - small volume pulse is seen in low cardiac output states
  - large volume—anaemia or other causes of hyperdynamic circulation, aortic regurgitation, patent ductus arteriosus, or other rarer systemic to pulmonary connections
- character (describes the waveform of the pulse):
  - slow rising and plateau—moderate or severe aortic stenosis
  - collapsing pulse—aortic incompetence, patent ductus arteriosus
  - pulsus paradoxus—pulse is weaker or disappears on inspiration, e.g. constrictive pericarditis, tamponade, status asthmaticus
  - jerky pulse—normal volume, rapidly rising and ill sustained; suggestive of hypertrophic cardiomyopathy or supravalvar aortic stenosis
- symmetry.

Blood pressure

- This can be done at the end but always mention it during the examination.
- The convention is to measure blood pressure in the right arm in a calm but awake subject. If conditions differ from this, they should be documented with the reading.
- Record the blood pressure in the left arm in case of peripheral vascular access in the right arm and in both arms and legs in suspected coarctation of the aorta or after Blalock–Taussig shunt and aortic surgery.
- Generally, the cuff bladder should cover at least two-thirds of the arm and three-quarters of the circumference.
- Estimate the systolic blood pressure initially by inflating the cuff fully and then deflating slowly while palpating the radial pulse. Note the blood pressure at the point when the radial pulse returns. This is useful in infants and toddlers.
- Following this, record the blood pressure by the auscultatory method which is the more accurate measure. Place the diaphragm of the stethoscope over the brachial artery along the medial aspect of the distal arm below the edge of the cuff. Inflate the cuff to 30 mm above the palpatory systolic blood pressure and then deflate slowly at the rate of 2–3 mm Hg per second. Systolic blood pressure is recorded at the point when clear, repetitive tapping sounds are just heard. Diastolic blood pressure is recorded when the sounds disappear.
- Auscultatory estimation of blood pressure can be difficult in infants. In these cases, systolic pressure by palpation should be noted.
- To measure lower limb blood pressure, apply the cuff to the thigh and palpate the dorsalis pedis.
- Readings should take the state of the child into account and should be in comparison to normal values related to height and sex of child. Avoid taking a blood pressure from an agitated screaming child!

Oedema

- foot
- sacral if immobile
- facial/periorbital (after superior cavopulmonary connection surgery).

System examination

Inspection

Jugular venous pressure (figure 5.3)

- Assessment of jugular venous pressure is rarely important in the younger child. It is also difficult to obtain an accurate reading because of the short neck in children but can be measured easily in children older than 8 years.
- Ask the child to lie on the couch with the head and chest elevated to 45° and breathe quietly. The jugular venous pressure is assessed by measuring the vertical distance between the top of the jugular venous pulsations and the sternal angle (angle of Louis). In cases where the top of the jugular pulsations is not visible at 45°, increasing the reclining angle up to 90° can make the pulsations visible.
- Exert firm and sustained pressure on the right upper quadrant of the abdomen and look for hepatojugular reflex, that is elevation in the jugular venous pressure by 2–3 cm.

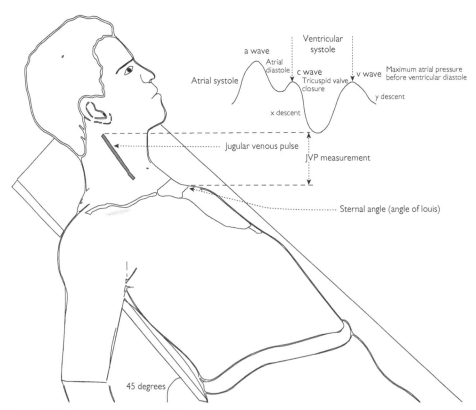

Figure 5.3 Jugular venous pressure (JVP).

- Jugular venous pressure is elevated in conditions such as right heart failure, fluid overload, and pericardial tamponade.

The chest (figure 5.4)

- Comment on the **shape of the chest**—whether it is symmetrical or asymmetrical. The following are some of the commonly seen abnormal shapes: pectus carinatum (pigeon chest), pectus excavatum (funnel chest), and Harrison's sulcus. Harrison's sulcus may occur in conditions with increased pulmonary blood flow, chronic or recurrent airway obstruction at any level including asthma, chronic lung disease, and rickets (figure 5.5).
- Look for **asymmetry of chest expansion.**
- The chest should be carefully inspected for **operative scars** (median sternotomy, lateral thoracotomy, drainage scars in epigastrium or subclavian/ axillary scars from pacemakers, vascular entry sites in neck and also in groin) and keloid.
- **Pulsations**—observe for apical impulse, parasternal, suprasternal, and epigastric pulsations. Apical impulse will be shifted downward and outward due to cardiomegaly and outward in collapse of the left lung or right pleural effusion.
- It is important to look for **scoliosis,** which can be easily missed. Look for scoliosis in the standing and not the sitting position.

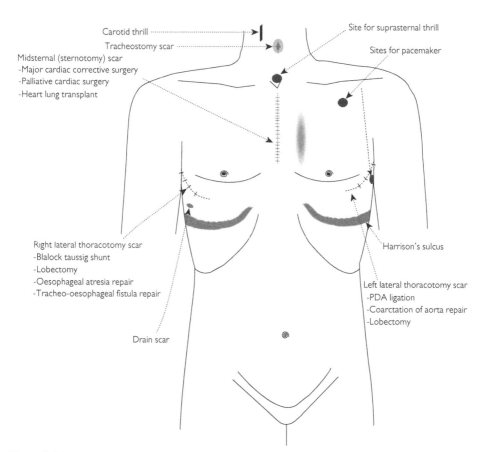

Figure 5.4 Inspection and palpation of the cardiovascular system.

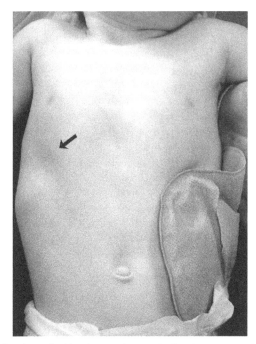

Figure 5.5 Harrison's sulcus (arrow) with colostomy bag attached to the stoma on the left side.

Palpation of the precordium

It is necessary to be gentle with palpation. *Ensure that your hands are warm for palpation.*

- **Apex or apical impulse** is the outermost and lowermost definite cardiac impulse on the chest wall. While describing the apical impulse, define its location and character. The apical impulse is normally felt in the fourth left intercostal space on the midclavicular line in most children but it may also be situated in the fifth intercostal space on the midclavicular line in older children. It can be displaced in cardiomegaly, scoliosis, and chest deformity. In dextrocardia, the apex will be on the right side; hence, always look for the apex on both sides of the chest. If dextrocardia is present, feel for the position of liver (situs inversus). Some children with cardiac disease have a midline liver. The quality of the apical impulse (determined by the thrust on the fingertip) can be sustained (aortic stenosis), forceful (left ventricular hypertrophy), or normal (figure 5.6).
- **Parasternal heave** is felt with the base of the palm in the supine position and is present in right ventricular hypertrophy.
- **Thrills** are palpable murmurs, best felt with the fingertips. While describing a thrill, mention its location and relationship to the cardiac cycle (e.g. systolic thrill at the left lower sternal edge). The presence of a thrill suggests the accompanying murmur is at least grade 4/6 in intensity. A carotid thrill may be present in aortic valvular stenosis.
- **Palpable pulmonary second heart sound** reflects pulmonary hypertension.

Percussion

Percussion has a limited role in the cardiovascular examination. It is useful in identifying a coexisting pleural effusion.

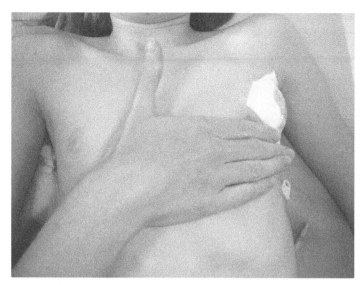

Figure 5.6 Palpation of the apex.

Auscultation (table 5.3)

Auscultation is a skill that needs plenty of practise. It is advisable to listen both with the bell and diaphragm in all areas. The bell must be applied to the chest wall lightly and is useful to auscultate low-pitched sounds such as the diastolic murmur of mitral stenosis and third heart sound. Various sounds from different heart valves are best heard at specific areas on the chest wall. Start at the apex (mitral area). After this, inch the stethoscope towards the left lower sternal edge (fourth left intercostal space, tricuspid area). Next, place the stethoscope at the left upper sternal edge, second left intercostal space (pulmonary area), and then at the right upper sternal edge, second right intercostal space (aortic area).

- Step 1: listen to the two components of the **first and second heart sounds** (S1, mitral and tricuspid valve closure, and S2, aortic and pulmonary valve closure). Comment on the loudness of S1 (normal, quiet in long PR interval and mitral regurgitation, loud in short PR interval and mitral stenosis). Report on the loudness of the aortic or pulmonary component (normally, aortic component is heard earlier and louder than pulmonary component, with the splitting well heard in inspiration but not in expiration), the presence of splitting (report it as 'single' if there is no split) and type of splitting (normal, wide, narrow, reversed, or fixed) (figure 5.7).
- Step 2: comment on the **presence or absence of extra heart sounds,** the S3 and S4. The **third heart sound** is a low-pitched, early diastolic sound, best heard at the apex with the bell. It is often heard as a gallop rhythm. The **fourth heart sound** is a late diastolic sound with a slightly higher pitch than S3. S4 is always pathological, while S3 is commonly heard in normal children.
- Step 3: listen for the presence of a **murmur** and comment accordingly. While describing a murmur, it is helpful to take the following approach:
  - where is the murmur in the cardiac cycle—systole or diastole—(a venous hum is the only normal systolo-diastolic murmur)?
  - where is it heard loudest on the precordium?
  - how is it best heard—using the bell or diaphragm?
  - loudness—commonly graded out of 6 (table 5.4)

Table 5.3 Heart sounds

Heart sound	Findings	Interpretation
1st heart sound	Loud 1st heart sound	Short PR interval Mechanical prosthetic atrioventricular valve Mitral stenosis
	Variable loudness of 1st heart sound	Heart block (quiet if PR long) Atrial fibrillation
2nd heart sound	Loud pulmonary 2nd sound	Pulmonary hypertension, increased pulmonary flow, e.g. PDA, ASD, large VSD
	Split 2nd sound	Wide and variable splitting: healthy normal children (widens in inspiration, aortic closure precedes pulmonary closure) Fixed splitting: ASD (no change with respiration) Wide splitting: ASD, pulmonary stenosis, right bundle branch block Reverse splitting (widens on expiration): left bundle branch block, severe aortic stenosis
	Single 2nd sound	Tetralogy of Fallot Severe pulmonary stenosis (inaudible pulmonary component) Transposition of great vessels Truncus arteriosus
3rd heart sound	Low pitched early diastolic sound, best heard over the apex	Normal in children Heart failure
4th heart sound	Late diastole, low pitched	Heart failure Pulmonary hypertension
Opening snap	Heard after 2nd heart sound, high pitched	Mitral stenosis
Ejection click	Heard after 1st heart sound, high pitched	Aortic or pulmonary valve stenosis (early systolic) Mitral valve prolapse— mid or late systolic click

ASD, atrial septal defect; ASD, atrial septal defect; PDA, patent ductus arteriosus.

- ◆ qualitative description—pitch and quality (high or low, harsh, blowing or rumbling)
- ◆ radiation (neck, axilla, sides, back) (table 5.5)
- ◆ changes with manoeuvre (dynamic auscultation)
  - ▪ lying and sitting position (venous hum disappears on lying down)
  - ▪ leaning forward: listen along the upper sternal edge, in an older cooperative child as they lean forward and breathe out, for early diastolic murmur of aortic regurgitation
  - ▪ respiration
  - ▪ valsalva.
- • Step 4: listen for **additional sounds** such as ejection click and opening snap.
- • Step 5: listen over the **suprasternal notch and carotids**. Loud radiation of systolic murmur to carotids suggests aortic stenosis. A quiet systolic bruit in the supraclavicular area and base of the neck, but not at the base of the heart, is a normal finding in healthy children.

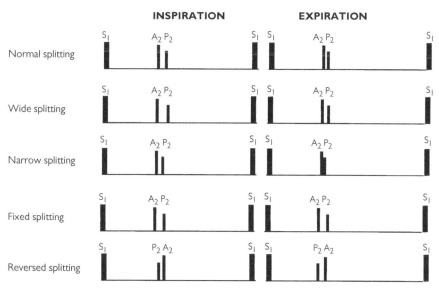

Figure 5.7 Normal, wide, narrow, fixed, and reverse splitting of the second heart sound.

Table 5.4 Grading of murmurs

Grade 1	Just audible by an expert in ideal conditions
Grade 2	Quiet; just heard by a non-expert in ideal conditions
Grade 3	Moderately loud
Grade 4	Loud with a palpable thrill
Grade 5	Very loud over a wide area with a palpable thrill
Grade 6	Audible with stethoscope off the chest or even without a stethoscope

- Step 6: last, but not the least, always listen at the **back**.
- In addition, depending on the case, it is useful to auscultate elsewhere:
  - head, for intracranial bruits
  - any vascular swelling (thyroid, liver, limb).

Other systems

Before completing the cardiac examination, it is important to look for the following:

- auscultation of the lungs
- abdomen—inspect for gastrostomy and palpate for hepatosplenomegaly
- offer to measure the oxygen saturation.

Table 5.5 Site and radiation of murmurs

Cause	Primary site	Radiation
Ventricular septal defect	Pansystolic systolic murmur at left sternal edge (4th left intercostal space, murmur present throughout systole)	All over precordium
Atrial septal defect	Ejection systolic murmur at left upper sternal border (2nd left intercostal space)	Radiates to back (to lung fields)
Pulmonary stenosis	Ejection systolic murmur at left upper sternal border (2nd left intercostal space)	Radiates towards left clavicle or back beneath left scapula (to lung fields)
Aortic stenosis	Ejection systolic murmur at right upper sternal border (2nd right intercostal space)	Radiates into the neck
Aortic regurgitation	Early diastolic murmur at left upper sternal edge	Down left sternal edge towards apex
Tricuspid regurgitation	Pansystolic murmur at lower left sternal edge	Lower right sternal edge, liver
Mitral regurgitation	Pansystolic murmur at apex	Left axilla, beneath left scapula
Mitral stenosis	Mid-diastolic murmur at apex	Does not radiate
Patent ductus arteriosus	Continuous murmur below left clavicle	Radiated to the back
Coarctation of the aorta	Systolic murmur between scapulae	Left sternal edge
Venous hum	Continuous murmur heard below the clavicles	Normal finding; disappears on lying the child down and elevating the legs
Pericardial friction rub	Creaking sound like walking on firm snow, best heard at left sternal border when breath is held	

Videos

Video 5.1 The cardiovascular examination is shown in the video by Dr Nick Archer, Consultant Paediatric Cardiologist from Oxford. You will notice that this is an extensive teaching session which goes beyond what would normally be expected from a candidate taking the exam. It clearly identifies all relevant aspects of the examination, which include establishing rapport and he gives a running commentary as he goes along. It is a well-structured, fluent, and systematic examination. He summarizes his findings and gives his interpretation.

Video 5.2 In the live candidate examination on a cardiovascular case, Dr Serane *deliberately* makes errors that are commonly made by candidates. These mistakes include poor rapport, bad examination technique, inconsistent findings, and poor interpretation. This is obviously an extreme example of a poorly performing candidate, which was created for demonstration purposes only and the mum was aware of the scenario. Please notice that it is easy to make a child uncooperative if one is not sensitive to the child's needs as shown in this station.

Chapter 6 **Examination of the respiratory system**

The examination of the respiratory system causes much anxiety among candidates, as many feel the findings are difficult to elicit, particularly in a small child. Just like other systems, having a structured approach makes identification and interpretation of the findings easy. It is important to practise the proper examination technique repeatedly, as this is the best way to improve the skills that are essential to obtain accurate findings. *However, the examination itself can be performed in a different sequence depending on the age and the degree cooperation of the child.*

The examination of the respiratory system is best done in correlation with the available medical history. First, assimilate the available history, which will give an idea of the expected findings and subsequent diagnosis. At the end of the examination, it is important to describe significant findings (table 6.1) with reference to specific surface locations, as shown in figure 6.1.

Key competence skills required in examination of the respiratory system are given in table 6.2.

General approach

These steps are repeated in every system to reiterate their importance and to help you recollect the initial approach of any clinical exam. Also refer to chapter 4.

- *On entering the examination room, demonstrate your strict adherence to infection control measures by washing your hands or by using alcohol rub.*
- Introduce yourself *both* to the parents and the child.
- Talk slowly and clearly with a smile on your face.
- Establish rapport with the child and parents.
- Expose the chest adequately while ensuring their privacy.
- Positioning the patient: the child should be undressed appropriately to the waist to allow proper examination. It may be easier to examine an older child when they sit on the edge of the bed, or on a chair. It is preferable to examine younger children on their parent's lap rather than on a couch separated from the parents, as this can cause much anxiety. Removing a toddler or an infant from his or her parent will most probably yield a screaming child in whom eliciting any physical findings will be virtually impossible.

Visual survey—head to toe examination

Start with a visual survey (inspection) from head to toe. It sounds impressive and professional if you narrate while examining the child. This approach has multiple advantages—it keeps everybody (particularly the examiner) engaged, you sound professional, the examiner knows what you are looking for, the atmosphere is lively, and you are less likely to miss out findings when summarizing at the end. Most importantly, this approach tells the examiner that you are 'thinking fast on your feet', which is what they are looking for. It is essential to *keep your hands off the child for as long as possible.* Comment on the following:

- look—general:
  - state of wakefulness: awake/ aware/ alert/ active
  - general well-being: well/ ill looking
  - position
  - interest in the surroundings: a sick child will not show any interest
  - size and appearance of the child: thin and small, thin and tall, well nourished and tall, well nourished and short. *Always make a comment that you would like to plot the child's height and weight on the growth chart.*
- look—specific:
  - pink in air or cyanosed

Table 6.1 Comparison of the clinical signs in common respiratory disorders

Sign	Consolidation	Collapse	Pleural effusion	Pneumothorax	Airflow obstruction	Bronchiectasis
Clubbing	Absent	Absent	Absent	Absent	Absent	May be present
Audible noise	Absent	Absent	Absent	Absent	Wheeze may be present	Absent
Work of breathing	May be increased	May be increased	May be increased	Often increased	May be increased	May be increased
Shape of the chest	Normal	May be flattened on the affected side	Normal	Normal	Harrison's sulcus ±	Harrison's sulcus ±
Tracheal/ apex beat position	Normal	Shifted to affected side	Shifted to less affected or normal side	Shifted to less affected or normal side	Normal	Normal unless associated collapse
Chest expansion	May be asymmetrical	May be asymmetrical	May be asymmetrical	May be asymmetrical	Usually symmetrical	Usually symmetrical
Percussion	Impaired	Impaired	Stony dull	Hyper-resonant	Usually normal	Usually normal
Breath sounds intensity	Reduced	Reduced	Markedly decreased	Decreased	Usually normal	Usually normal unless associated collapse
Breath sounds quality	Bronchial sounds	Bronchial sounds (if bronchus is unobstructed)	Normal	Normal	Normal (prolonged expiration)	Bronchial sounds
Added sounds	Crackles +++	Crackles ±	Crackles ± (in collapsed lung above fluid)	None	Wheeze (mono- or polyphonic)	Crackles ± wheeze (occasional)
Vocal resonance	Aegophony	Reduced	Reduced	Normal or reduced	Normal	Normal
Dynamic auscultation	Post-tussive crackles ±	Post-tussive crackles ±	None	None	Post-tussive wheeze	Post-tussive crackles +
Peak flow	–	–	–	–	Decreased	–

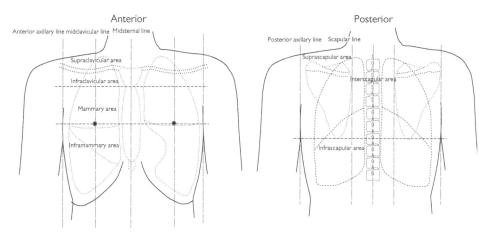

Figure 6.1 Landmarks of the chest.

Table 6.2 Key competence skills required in examination of the respiratory system

Competence skill	Standard
Knowledge of descriptive terms used in respiratory examination	Ability to use the correct terminology for findings
Understanding of correct positioning of the patient	Position the patient correctly and adequately expose the chest
Adequate knowledge, clear understanding, and ability to detect and interpret clinical features of the respiratory system examination	Demonstrate a systematic approach to the respiratory system examination, including inspection, palpation, percussion, and auscultation
	Ability to elicit signs accurately, interpret these signs correctly, and make appropriate conclusions
	Demonstrate understanding of the use of peak expiratory flow rate to assess respiratory function, especially in children with reactive airway disease, and interpret a peak flow diary
Ability to summarize findings, offer a differential diagnosis, and discuss a management plan	Demonstrate ability to describe findings in a cohesive manner and offer an appropriate differential diagnosis
	Demonstrate ability to offer a suitable management plan

- ◆ head:
  - ▪ size: microcephaly, macrocephaly
  - ▪ shape: dolichocephaly (seen in ex-preterm infants)
- ◆ face: normal or dysmorphic features (using the word 'dysmorphic' can be offensive to some parents; instead describe what you see)
- ◆ conjunctiva (palpebral and bulbar)
- ◆ mouth: halitosis, seen in bronchiectasis
- ◆ mucous membrane (tongue): colour (pallor, cyanosis, jaundice), ulcers, candidiasis (cyanosis is easily missed if pink curtains surround the child's bed)
- ◆ teeth: look for the presence of teeth (age appropriate), dental caries, or abnormal teeth
- ◆ tonsils: inflamed, pustular exudate on tonsils (tonsillitis)
- ◆ pharynx: red and inflamed (pharyngitis)

- nose: nasal polyp, deviated septum (nasal obstruction), swollen turbinates (allergies); make a comment about palpating sinuses for tenderness (sinusitis) but *don't* do this as it will be painful to the child.
- skin: associated disease such as eczema, engorged superficial veins in superior vena caval obstruction, subcutaneous emphysema
- hands and nails: pallor, peripheral cyanosis, single palmar crease (trisomy 21), clubbing (seen in cystic fibrosis and bronchiectasis, refer to chapter 5)
- sputum: colour, amount, consistency, blood, purulence
- equipment: oxygen mask, nasal cannula, intravenous catheter, pulse oximeter, feeding tube, gastrostomy, nebulizer, peak flow meter, sputum cup, physiotherapy aids, medications such as Creon (pancrelipase capsules) in cystic fibrosis
- **respiration**—while examining for respiratory movements, comment on the following:
  - rate: in the exam, you can count the rate for 15 seconds and multiply by four, but tell the examiner that, ideally, you would like to count for 1 minute; increase in respiration can be physiological (exercise, anxiety) or pathological (fever, disease of lung and heart, metabolic conditions such as acidosis)
  - rhythm: respiration is normally regular; normal infants can have periodic breathing characterized by brief pauses in breathing lasting for a few seconds
  - type of breathing: in children, the respiration is mainly abdominal and is similar to that seen in adult males; presence of thoracic breathing in a child is indicative of intra-abdominal pathology
  - degree of breathlessness: none, mild (chest recession), or severe (chest recession, use of sternocleidomastoid and nasal flaring)
  - duration of expiratory phase: comment on the duration of expiration, which is prolonged in obstructive airway disease such as asthma
- listen:
  - voice: comment on hoarseness—seen in laryngitis and recurrent laryngeal nerve palsy
  - noise:
    - wheeze suggests bronchospasm; it could be due to bronchial asthma or chronic lung disease
    - stridor is caused by obstruction of the larynx, trachea or large airways; it is a croaking noise, loudest on inspiration and could be due to stenosis, laryngitis, or a foreign body
    - grunting is due to expiration against a closed glottis
    - cough: lack of explosive beginning may point to vocal cord paralysis ('bovine' cough); wheezy cough suggests bronchial asthma; loose productive cough suggests excessive bronchial secretions; dry cough may occur with lower respiratory tract infection, asthma, chronic lung disease, and heart failure (table 6.3).

Tactile examination—general

- pulse:
  - brachial pulse in an infant and toddler, radial in older children (refer to chapter 5)
  - check both the right and left sides
  - rate: tachycardia (asthma, severe respiratory illness)
  - pulsus paradoxus (commonly seen in severe asthma)
- blood pressure can be done at the end of the examination, but should be mentioned during the examination
- axilla: lymph nodes
- neck: lymph nodes, thyroid swelling, venous pulse.

Table 6.3 Different types of cough and their significance

Type	Significance
Dry, nocturnal cough	Chronic pharyngitis, tracheitis, laryngitis, psychological
Barking cough	Acute laryngotracheobronchitis, spasmodic croup
Brassy cough	High-pitched cough caused by irritation of the vagus nerve
Honking cough	Psychological
Paroxysmal cough with a whoop	Pertussis
Croupy cough	Harsh, barking, dry cough similar to a seal barking, seen in laryngotracheobronchitis
Wet cough	Due to secretions in the respiratory tract, seen in lower respiratory tract infections

System examination

Both anterior and posterior aspects of the chest should be examined. Examine the front before going to the back—this is more comfortable for the patient and you look impressive. Always compare the right with the left side during examination.

Inspection of the chest (figure 6.2)

Satisfactory exposure of the chest is essential to avoid missing some important signs. However, it is important to be careful while exposing older and adolescent girls, with whom limited exposure should be practised. Make sure that when the child is undressed the curtains are drawn, irrespective of the child's age.

The child should be examined ideally in the sitting position in daylight rather than artificial light. Inspection should be carried out from four directions.

- ◆ front
- ◆ from both sides; this is useful for identifying anteroposterior diameter and kyphosis
- ◆ from behind
- ◆ from above downwards.

If the child is lying down, inspection should be carried out from the foot end of the bed, from the top (directly over the patient) and then from the sides, making sure to get down to the level of the child.

- Shape of the chest: the chest is cylindrical in children, hence the anteroposterior and lateral diameters are nearly equal. In pectus carinatum, the sternum bulges forward with straightening of the anterior ribs and the chest is triangular in shape. In pectus excavatum, the depressed sternum produces a funnel-shaped chest anteriorly. Harrison's sulcus is the linear depression of the lower ribs just above the costal margin on both sides and is seen in chronic respiratory disorders, poorly controlled asthma, chronic congestive cardiac failure, and rickets in infants and toddlers.
- Symmetry of the chest: asymmetry of the chest can be a result of spinal deformity or flattening (loss of lung volume) or bulging of the chest wall.
- Chest movement: expansion of the upper lobes is best assessed by inspection from behind the patient, looking down the clavicles during moderate respiration. For assessment of lower lobe expansion, the chest should be inspected posteriorly. While examining chest movement, look at the depth and symmetry of the breathing movements.

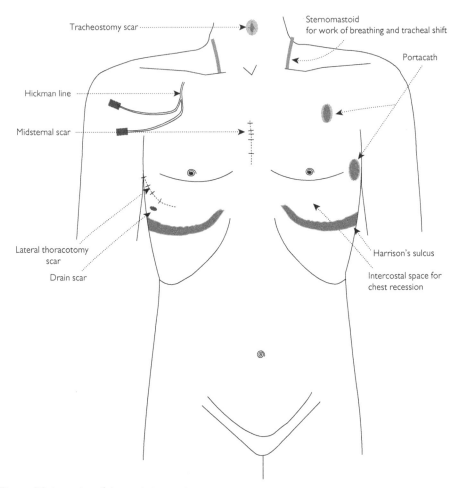

Figure 6.2 Inspection of the respiratory system.

- Work of breathing: can be assessed by looking for the following:
  - excessive working of the sternomastoid muscles
  - intercostal and subcostal recession
  - sternal recession
  - paradoxical movement of the chest and abdomen (see-saw breathing)
  - flaring of the ala nasi
  - grunting.
- Sputum: observe colour, amount, consistency, purulence, blood.
- Scars: midsternal, thoracotomy (do not miss the posterolateral ones, particularly in a lying child), tracheostomy, and drain scars (refer to chapter 5).
- Local swellings and oedema of the chest wall.
- Devices:
  - intravenous access devices: Hickman line and Portacath
  - inhalational medication delivery devices

- ◆ sputum cup
- ◆ Creon tablets.
- Neck:
  - ◆ Trail's sign: prominence of the clavicular head of the sternomastoid on the side of tracheal displacement
  - ◆ raised jugular venous pressure suggests right heart failure or superior vena caval obstruction.
- Spine: look for kyphoscoliosis.

Palpation

Before palpating the child, warm your hands by rubbing them against each other to avoid discomfort to the child. Also, ask the child about painful areas before continuing with the examination; examine those areas at the end, gently. While examining the front of the chest, the child's upper extremities should be by their side. Ask the child to keep both hands above the head while examining the axilla. Ask the child to lean forward and cross their arms in front of the chest to get the scapula out of the way for palpation, percussion, and auscultation of back. The scheme for palpation of the chest should include:

- Mediastinal position:
  - ◆ Tracheal position: be gentle and explain clearly what you are going to do, as some children can otherwise feel threatened. Keep the middle finger on the notch, the index finger on one side and the ring finger on the other side and look for deviation. Deviated trachea usually indicates an upper lobe problem. Slight deviation of the trachea to the right is often normal.
  - ◆ Apex beat (refer to chapter 5): might be shifted because of kyphoscoliosis or depressed sternum or cardiomegaly. The mediastinum will be 'pushed away' by pleural effusion and pneumothorax and 'pulled towards' by collapse and less commonly, fibrosis. Consolidation does not change the mediastinal position.
- Chest expansion: it is possible to assess the chest expansion by palpation in children older than 5 years. During palpation, compare the chest expansion on one side with the opposite side. In general, the side with lesser movement is the diseased side. Assessment of chest expansion is carried out from above downwards, initially anteriorly and then posteriorly. Place the hands symmetrically on the chest with the thumbs meeting in the midline and observe the thumb movement away from midline on deep inspiration (figure 6.3).
- Tracheal tug: place the middle finger on the trachea; in the presence of tug, the trachea moves inferiorly with each inspiration. It points to a marked increase in the work of breathing.
- Vocal fremitus: this sign is the palpation of the vibrations caused by phonation. Place the ulnar border of the hand and ask the child to say 'ninety-nine' again and again, with the same tone and intensity. Compare the vibrations on corresponding areas. Vocal fremitus is increased in consolidation (with a patent bronchus) and decreased in effusion or pneumothorax. This crude sign has been superseded by vocal resonance and *it is not usually performed in the examination*.
- Crepitus: crackling sensation felt on palpating the skin of the chest or neck. It is seen in subcutaneous emphysema.

Percussion

Percussion is useful both for the identification of underlying lung disease and the borders of the lungs, liver, and heart. Percussion is best performed in a quiet room with the child either sitting or standing. Place the middle finger (pleximeter) of the non-dominant hand on the area to be percussed. Strike the back of the middle phalanx of the pleximeter with the tip of the middle finger of the other hand (the plexor) at 90°, with movement delivered mainly from the wrist rather than elbow. *The blow should be just hard enough to elicit the resonance and once struck, lift the finger immediately* (figure 6.4).

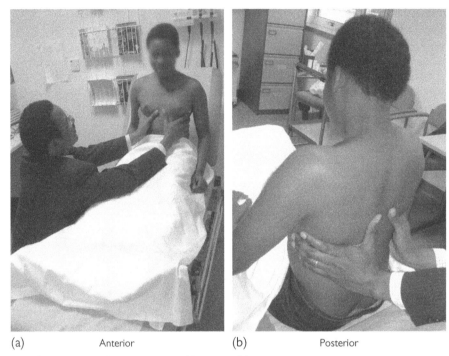

(a)   Anterior   (b)   Posterior

Figure 6.3 Assessment of chest movement; (a) anterior, (b) posterior.

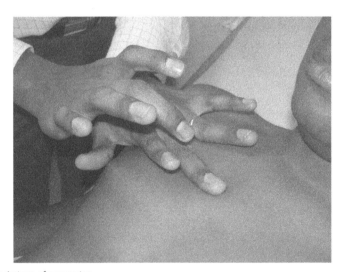

Figure 6.4 Technique of percussion.

While percussing the clavicle, the bone acts as the pleximeter and so percuss on the bone directly. The areas to be percussed are clavicle, three anterior (supraclavicular area, mammary, and inframammary areas), axilla (axillary and infra-axillary area), and three posterior (suprascapular, interscapular, and infrascapular areas) (figure 6.5). While percussing for the borders of organs, the pleximeter should be parallel to the border to be identified.

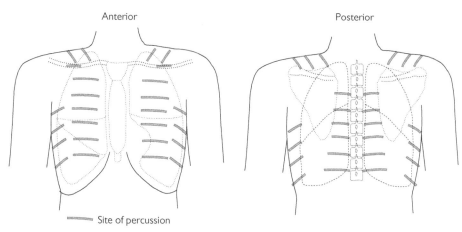

Figure 6.5 Sites for chest percussion.

- increased resonance—hard to detect, seen in pneumothorax
- impaired resonance—collapse consolidation
- stony dullness—effusion.

Common errors of percussion
- placing the entire hand on the chest instead of the pleximeter finger alone
- fulcrum of the percussing movement from elbow rather than wrists
- striking either too vigorously or too softly
- percussing one entire lung and then moving to the other lung instead of comparing both sides at every level
- not asking the child to cross their arms across their chest to move the scapula laterally while percussing posteriorly.

Auscultation

Auscultation helps to confirm the findings identified by the preceding examination techniques and, sometimes, it may be the only way of recognizing new findings. Always auscultate on the skin and not over the patient's gown or clothing. Ask the child (if old enough to understand) to 'breath in and out, through the mouth, in their own time'. Infants and toddlers are best auscultated when they are quiet. While auscultating posteriorly, ask the child to cross their arms in front of their chest. Listen for an entire respiratory cycle at every location. *Do not* move the stethoscope while the patient is breathing out.

- Intensity of the breath sounds: it is better to describe intensity than to speak about air entry. The latter is a physical phenomenon, which cannot be measured by listening to breath sounds alone. Reduced breath sounds are present in pneumonia, pleural effusion, pneumothorax, and collapse.
- Prolongation of the expiratory phase is seen, for example, in obstructive airway disease.
- Be able to recognize abnormal character of the breath sounds like bronchial breath sound which is different to normal from vesicular breath sounds. Vesicular breath sounds are louder and longer in inspiration than expiration and there is no gap between the inspiratory and expiratory phase. Bronchial breath sounds have a hollow, blowing quality and are audible throughout expiration. There is a gap between inspiration and expiration. Bronchial breath sound is audible normally just below the neck posteriorly and the right upper chest where the trachea is contiguous with the right main bronchus. It is also heard over areas of consolidation, collapse with unobstructed airway, bronchiectasis, and fibrosis.

- Be able to recognize and describe added sounds (crepitations, wheezes), their nature and timing (e.g. end expiratory crackles). Wheezes are continuous musical sounds, louder in expiration than inspiration. A wheeze suggests significant airway narrowing and can be absent in severe airway obstruction due to lack of airflow. Crackles are interrupted sounds, non-musical in nature, and suggest loss of stability of smaller airways (early inspiratory) or alveolar disease (throughout or end inspiratory). They can be heard with pneumonia, bronchiectasis (coarse, gurgling), or left ventricular failure (fine).
- Vocal resonance:
  - Ask the child to say 'ninety-nine' while listening to each part of chest.
  - Muffled is normal.
  - Clearly heard speech (aegophony) means consolidation.
  - Markedly reduced sounds suggest effusion or collapse with obstructed bronchus.
- Dynamic auscultation:
  - following cough.

Common errors during auscultation
- auscultating over the clothing
- auscultating one entire lung and then moving to the other lung instead of comparing both sides at every level
- not beginning the auscultation at the apex of lungs
- hastily moving the stethoscope before exhalation is complete.

Other examination techniques

- Peak flow in children older than 6 years: ask the child to take a full breath in and exhale rapidly through the mouth into the PEFR meter. Normal value depends on age, sex, and height. Airway obstruction results in reduced and variable PEFR.
- Inhaler technique.

Other systems

- Abdomen: palpate for hepatomegaly (increased liver span) or pushed down liver of obstructive lung disease (normal liver span but palpable below the costal margin).
- Cardiovascular examination: to rule out signs of right heart failure or associated underlying cardiac illness.
- The ENT examination is part of the respiratory examination and therefore, should be examined (or at least you should offer to do so).

After examining the child wash hands or disinfect hands with alcohol gel.

Video

Video 6.1 In this video, Dr O'Keeffe examines the respiratory system of child. Note his technique for examining an uncooperative child. He identifies all relevant aspects of the examination and gives a running commentary as he goes along. It is a well-structured, fluent, and systematic examination. He summarizes and interprets his findings.

Chapter 7 **Examination of the abdomen**

The examination of the abdomen is one of the easier cases in the clinical exam. It is, however, easy for candidates to fail this station if they cannot elicit the appropriate physical findings. As always, listen carefully to the examiner's instructions. You may be asked to examine either the gastrointestinal system or only the abdomen; they are not the same. Occasionally, you may be instructed to palpate the abdomen and beginning at the hands in such situations will annoy the examiner. While giving instructions to the child, you must use simple language that can be easily understood. The examination of the abdomen is best done in correlation with the available medical history, as it often gives major clues. It helps to have a systematic approach to presenting your findings, which should be practised thoroughly. However, the examination process itself can be performed in a different sequence depending on the age of the child and their degree of cooperation.

Key competence skills required in the examination of the abdomen are given in table 7.1. Abdominal cases commonly encountered in the MRCPCH Clinical Exam are listed in table 7.2.

General approach

These are repeated in every system to reiterate their importance and to help you recollect the initial approach of any clinical exam. Also refer to chapter 4.

- *On entering the examination room, demonstrate your adherence to infection control measures by washing your hands or decontaminating them using alcohol rub.*
- Introduce yourself *both* to the parents and the child.
- Talk slowly and clearly with a smile on your face.
- Establish rapport with the child and parents (remember that ignoring the child can have negative consequences!).

Table 7.1 Key competence skills required in the examination of the abdomen

Competence skill	Standard
Knowledge of appropriate descriptive terms used for clinical findings of the abdomen	Demonstrate understanding that the abdomen is divided into nine regions for descriptive purposes
	Ability to use the correct terminology for findings
Understanding the importance of correct positioning of the child	Demonstrate ability to position the patient correctly
Knowledge and clear understanding of how to carry out a complete abdominal examination	Demonstrate a systematic approach of abdominal examination—inspection, palpation, percussion, and auscultation
	Elicit clinical signs and recognize associated abnormalities
	Awareness that the genitalia and rectum may need to be examined as clinically indicated, but this is not appropriate in the MRCPCH exam
Inspection	Ability to perform a general inspection including the hands, head and neck, and the abdomen
Palpation	Demonstrate ability to detect hepatomegaly, splenomegaly, enlarged kidneys, and presence of masses
Percussion	Ability to percuss for shifting dullness, liver span, and urinary bladder
Auscultation	Demonstrate ability to auscultate for bowel sounds, hepatic, splenic, and renal bruit
Summarize findings, offer a differential diagnosis and discuss a management plan	Demonstrate ability to describe findings and offer a possible differential diagnosis list (see tables 7.3, 7.4, and 7.5)
	Offer an appropriate management plan

Table 7.2 Abdominal conditions that may be seen in the MRCPCH Clinical Exam

Cause	Disease
Congenital	Umbilical hernia in Beckwith–Wiedemann syndrome
	Prune belly syndrome
Inflammatory	Inflammatory bowel disease
	Crohn's disease
	Ulcerative colitis
Metabolic/ miscellaneous	Failure to thrive (FTT)
	Malabsorption
	Short gut syndrome
	Cystic fibrosis
	Chronic renal failure

- Ensure privacy: to expose the abdomen adequately, the child should be undressed to the waist. Be careful when exposing older children and adolescents, with whom limited exposure should be practised. Cover the lower part of the body with a bed sheet, to avoid accidental exposure.
- Positioning: initial inspection may be done in the standing position. Growth, nutrition, hernias, and abdominal distension are best evaluated in this position. Further examination is carried out with the child lying down on their back comfortably, with a pillow supporting the head, hands at the sides, and legs uncrossed. Examine infants and toddlers on their parent's lap. Removing a toddler from their parents is less likely to yield good clinical signs and more likely to yield a screaming child.

Visual survey—head to toe examination

As always, start with inspection from head to toe and then proceed to tactile examination from the hands onwards. Remember the basic rule of 'looking at the patient and describing without touching'. Also, it might be better if you give a running commentary throughout the examination. When the examiner asks you to perform a specific task such as palpate the abdomen, first describe the general condition of the child in a nut shell.

Comment on the following: *look carefully and observe*

- state of wakefulness
- general well being: well or ill-looking child
- resting position
- interest in the surroundings
- size of the child: *comment that you would like to plot the child's height and weight on the growth chart*; if the examiner asks you to plot, make sure that you have the appropriate growth chart for the age and sex of the child; *assessment of the nutritional status of the child is very important in the context of the abdominal examination*
- employ the Tanner's developmental stages provided on standard growth charts to assess adolescents
- race is particularly relevant in the abdominal examination; for example sickle cell disease is common in Afro-Caribbean people and the spleen may be palpable in the younger but not in the older child
- environment (equipment): oxygen mask, nasal cannula, intravenous catheter, feeding tube, gastrostomy, feeding pump, medications (Creon in cystic fibrosis), nappies in older children, urinary catheter, etc.

- pink or pale in air
- head: size, shape
- face: haemolytic facies is seen in chronic haemolytic anaemia, such as thalassaemia due to extramedullary haematopoiesis
- conjunctiva: palpebral and bulbar
- hydration status
- mouth: ulcers are seen in Crohn's disease, pigmentation in Peutz–Jeghers syndrome, large tongue in hypothyroidism, Beckwith–Wiedemann syndrome, glycogen storage disease, and Down's syndrome
- teeth: dental caries
- tonsils and pharynx
- hands and nails: koilonychia suggests iron deficiency; clubbing of fingers may occur with inflammatory bowel disease and cystic fibrosis
- skin: scratch marks, bruises, petechiae, café-au-lait spots, skin nodules, scars
- signs of liver failure: asterixis (flapping tremor), palmar erythema, gynaecomastia, spider naevi.

General tactile examination

Pulse

- brachial pulse in an infant or toddler, radial in an older child
- check both right and left side (refer to chapter 5).

Blood pressure

Blood pressure may be measured at the end of the examination or at least mention that you would like to measure this. Hypertension may be present in neurofibromatosis, renal artery stenosis, and in some abdominal tumours such as pheochromocytomas.

System examination

Examination of the abdomen has two components, namely, **anterior abdominal examination** and **examination of posterior aspect of the abdomen**. Complete the anterior abdominal examination before moving to the back. Findings on the anterior aspect can be described based on quadrants (right upper quadrant, right lower quadrant, left upper quadrant, left lower quadrant) or nine regions.

Inspection

Adequate exposure of the abdomen is essential to ensure that the signs are not missed. The lighting should be good for inspection of the abdomen. As discussed earlier, the initial inspection should be carried out in the standing position, which makes it easier to identify global distension, hernia, and distended veins. Further inspection and examination can be carried in the supine position (figures 7.1 and 7.2).

- **Shape**: the abdominal contour can be scaphoid, flat, or distended. Symmetrical distension of the abdomen may be due to fat, faeces, fluid (ascites), flatus, or fetus (less likely)—the so called five Fs.
- **Symmetry** of the abdomen: altered in local visceroptosis (where organs may be displaced from their natural position) or paralysis of the abdominal muscle. Divarication of recti may be seen in hypotonia or after prolonged abdominal distension.
- **Skin**: look for scars, striae, stoma, or rashes. A linear scar suggests previous surgery. Multiple needle scars are indicative of medication administration (insulin in diabetics, desferrioxamine in haemolytic anaemia). Striae can be seen in obesity or postpregnancy state.

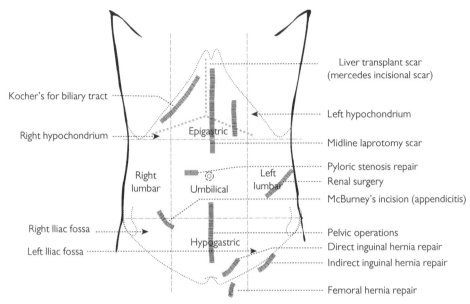

Figure 7.1 Inspection of the abdomen—quadrants and scar sites.

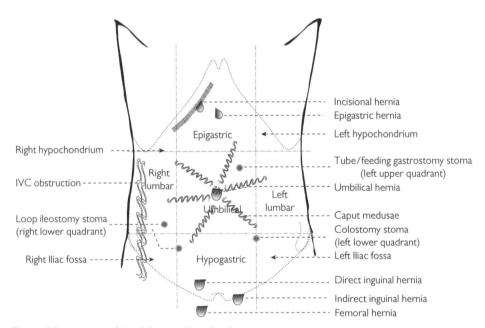

Figure 7.2 Inspection of the abdomen—hernial and stoma sites.

- **Umbilicus**: normal umbilicus is either flat or depressed. Careful examination for discharge is necessary, as it indicates underlying patent urachus or fistula. Presence of granulation tissue suggests umbilical granuloma.
- **Respiratory movements**: look for movement of the abdomen with respiration. Diminished movement is seen in guarding of muscles (peritonitis). Paradoxical movement (abdomen moving in with inspiration) is seen in bilateral diaphragmatic paralysis.
- **Peristaltic movements**: these can be visible in thin or malnourished children. Apart from these conditions, visible gastric peristalsis (movement from left hypochondrium towards the umbilicus and then to the right) is seen in pyloric stenosis, while visible intestinal peristalsis (movement from right to left and usually below or at the level of the umbilicus) is seen in intestinal obstruction. It is highly unlikely that any surgical abdomen will be used as a case in the exam.
- **Veins**: distended veins are normally not seen over the abdomen and, when present, indicate portal hypertension or inferior vena cava obstruction.
- **Hernia**: this is seen as a localized lump of variable size. Small hernias are better felt than seen, usually when the child is coughing or crying. Hernias arise due to weakness in the abdominal wall, which evolves into a localized defect. Weakening can be congenital or due to connective tissue problems (Ehlers–Danlos syndrome, Marfan's syndrome), scars from previous surgery or chronic increase in intra-abdominal pressure. The common abdominal hernias are:
  - inguinal hernia (congenital weakness at the internal inguinal ring or weak posterior wall of the inguinal canal)
  - femoral hernia (weak posterior wall of the femoral canal)
  - umbilical hernia (weakness at the site of insertion of the umbilical cord, more common in infants of African descent, ex-premature infants, and hypothyroidism; usually resolves spontaneously)
  - incisional hernia (weakness at the site of surgical incision)
  - epigastric hernia (through the linea alba above the umbilicus)
  - lumbar hernia (hernia in the lumbar region).
- **Genitalia**: mention that inspection of the genitalia would be necessary to complete a full examination, but do not do so in the exam unless the examiner specifically instructs you to.

Palpation

Palpation provides maximum information in an abdominal examination and is best done in the supine position. In older children with a firm abdomen, support the neck with a pillow and partially flex the legs at the hips and knees to relax the abdominal muscles. A pillow under the knees may also aid relaxation of abdominal muscles. While palpating the abdomen, *your hand and forearm should be in the same plane as the abdominal wall*. To achieve this, *get down to the level of the child*, either by kneeling down next to the bed or sitting on a low chair. Warm your hands before placing them on the patient by rubbing them against each other to avoid reflex muscle contraction and discomfort to the child. Keep your hands supple with fingers slightly flexed for easy and effective palpation. Never forget to ask the child '*does it hurt anywhere?*' Don't cause pain to the child in your anxiety when palpating the abdomen. Even for deep structures, palpation should be gentle. Start with the least painful area first, before proceeding to the more tender areas. *Always look at the child's face for any signs of discomfort*. In obese children, reinforce the hand on the abdominal surface by placing the other hand over it. There are three stages of abdominal palpation:

1. Superficial palpation: this provides a general idea of tone of the abdominal wall and calms down the child.
2. Deep palpation: this is useful for identifying organ enlargement and masses.
3. Bimanual palpation: this is useful for palpating the kidneys.

- **State of the abdominal muscles**: look for guarding or rigidity of the muscles. Guarding is involuntary contraction of the abdominal muscles on stimulation, whereas rigidity is contraction of the abdominal muscles at rest (without any stimulation). These indicate the presence of peritoneal irritation (peritonitis).

- **Tenderness**: tenderness at any site usually indicates inflammation of the underlying organ. Press the abdomen with the finger tips and suddenly release the pressure. If the child feels pain on release, rebound tenderness is present and indicates inflammation of the underlying parietal peritoneum.
- **Liver** (figure 7.3):
  - ◆ Start at the right iliac fossa area. Ask the child to take deep breath and palpate with the fingers parallel to the costal margin and pointing upwards. Move the fingers upwards during expiration in stages until you reach the costal margin. Continue tracing the edge across the midline towards the left side to identify the extent of the left lobe of the liver. After defining the border, palpate the surface of liver and look for tenderness. Note the surface (smooth or nodular), consistency (firm, soft, hard), and presence of pulsation (pulsatile in arteriovenous malformation and expansile in tricuspid regurgitation).
  - ◆ Palpation of the liver edge below the costal margin can be due to hepatomegaly or pushed-down liver, which can be differentiated by measuring the liver span (table 7.3). Identify the upper margin of the liver by percussing deeply for a dull note along the midclavicular line from the fourth intercostal space with the pleximeter parallel to the ribs. Calculate the liver span by measuring the distance between the upper margin and the liver edge on the midclavicular line.
- **Spleen** (figure 7.4; tables 7.4 and 7.5):
  - ◆ Start from the right iliac fossa and move the palpating right hand diagonally towards the left hypochondriac area, as the child breathes in and out until you reach the tip of the 10th rib. On reaching the left upper quadrant, place your left hand around the lower left rib cage and palpate below the costal margin with your right hand. If the spleen is still not palpable, ask the child to roll onto the right side. This will bring the edge of the spleen forwards and makes it easier to palpate. A spleen is rarely palpable normally, except in infancy.
  - ◆ It is essential to differentiate a splenic mass from a renal mass. A spleen enlarges downwards and diagonally towards the right iliac fossa (crosses the midline). It moves well with respiration, has a notch on the medial side, one cannot get above it, and is dull to percussion (usually the splenic area of dullness extends over the 9th, 10th, and 11th ribs, behind posterior axillary line).

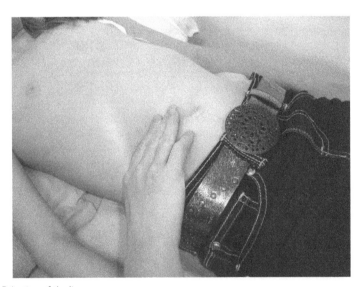

Figure 7.3 Palpation of the liver.

Table 7.3 Causes of hepatomegaly

Infections	Bacterial	Typhoid fever Tuberculosis Sepsis Cholangitis
	Viral	Viral hepatitis Viral (Epstein–Barr virus, cytomegalovirus) Acquired immune deficiency syndrome
	Parasitic	Amoebic liver abscess Echinococcal cysts Schistosomiasis Kala azar
Inflammatory		Juvenile idiopathic arthritis Systemic lupus erythematosus
Infiltrative		Metastasis Leukaemia Lymphoma Hepatoblastoma Histiocytosis
Congestive		Congestive heart failure Tricuspid stenosis/ regurgitation Constrictive pericarditis Budd–Chiari syndrome
Storage		Glycogen storage diseases Lipidoses (e.g. Niemann–Pick, Gaucher's disease) Mucopolysaccharidoses (e.g. Hurler's syndrome) Wilson's disease Porphyrias Haemochromatosis Fatty liver
Intrinsic		Cirrhosis
Structural		Biliary atresia Polycystic liver disorder Haemangioma
Metabolic		Hereditary fructose intolerance Galactosaemia Reye's syndrome Toxin exposure
Pushed down liver (palpable liver, no hepatomegaly)	Pulmonary	Asthma Bronchiolitis Pneumothorax
	Subdiaphragmatic	Subdiaphragmatic abscess

- **Kidneys** (figure 7.5): to palpate the right kidney, place your right hand over the right lumbar area and place your left hand posteriorly in the loin area. Ask the child to take slow and deep breaths. Push the right hand downwards towards the loin while pulling the left hand forwards (bimanual palpation). An enlarged kidney will be felt between the two hands. The left kidney can be palpated from the right side by leaning across the patient with the right hand over the left lumbar area and the left hand in the left loin posteriorly. Alternatively, the child can be examined from the left side with the right hand under the left loin and the left hand over the left lumbar area.

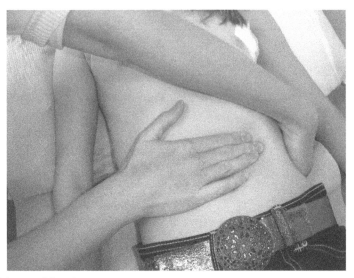

Figure 7.4 Palpation of the spleen.

Normal-sized kidneys are not usually palpable except in slim individuals. The kidney is bimanually palpable, ballottable, one can get above it, it is resonant to percussion (due to overlying colon), and does not move freely with respiration.

- **Mass**: if a mass is palpable, determine its characteristics, namely size, shape, surface, edge, consistency, tenderness, movement with respiration, pulsations, percussion note, and presence of bruit. A mass of pyloric stenosis becomes prominent while feeding (test feed).
- **Hernial orifices**: palpate all hernial sites (femoral, inguinal, umbilical orifices) at rest and during coughing for any evidence of hernia.
- **Fluid thrill**: ascites can be detected by using fluid thrill (massive ascites) or shifting dullness (moderate ascites). To elicit the fluid thrill, tap one flank and feel the transmitted wave on the opposite flank. Place another person's hand firmly on the midline to dampen vibrations conducted via fat. (The 'Puddle sign', which used to be performed, is no longer done, as it is inaccurate and causes discomfort to the child.)
- **Arterial pulsation**: aortic pulsation can normally be felt in thin children. It can also be felt in aortic aneurysm or when an overlying mass transmits the aortic pulsations. Pulsations are felt by pressing deeply in the midline, above the umbilicus. A well-defined, pulsatile mass, greater than 3 cm in diameter suggests an aortic aneurysm.
- **Determination of the direction of blood flow in distended veins**: occlude the vein with two adjacent fingers, empty it by massaging and spreading the fingers apart and then look for the direction of refill after removing the occlusion. In portal hypertension, veins radiate from the umbilicus (caput medusae) and blood flow is away from the umbilicus. In extrahepatic inferior vena caval obstruction, the blood flow in the distended veins is towards the umbilicus (figure 7.6).

Percussion

Percussion is useful for identifying the upper border of liver (to differentiate enlarged liver from pushed down liver), mild splenomegaly, and ascites and is best performed in a quiet room in the supine position. Place the middle finger (pleximeter) of the non-dominant hand on the part to be

Table 7.4 Causes of moderate splenomegaly

Infection	Bacterial	Subacute bacterial endocarditis Septicaemia Splenic abscess Typhoid fever Brucellosis Leptospirosis Tuberculosis Cat-scratch disease
	Viral	Acute viral hepatitis Viral (Epstein–Barr virus, cytomegalovirus) Acquired immune deficiency syndrome
	Parasitic	Toxoplasmosis Malaria Schistosomiasis Leishmaniasis Trypanosomiasis
	Fungal	Histoplasmosis
Inflammation/ disordered immunoregulation		Systemic lupus erythematosus Rheumatoid arthritis Inflammatory bowel disease Coeliac disease Chronic granulomatous disease Serum sickness Immune thrombocytopenia Drug reactions
Extramedullary haematopoiesis	Haemolytic anaemia	Hereditary spherocytosis Haemoglobinopathies Thalassaemia major Osteopetrosis (rare) Nutritional anaemias Marrow damage by radiation, toxins
Congestive	Portal hypertension	Splenic venous thrombosis Cirrhosis Portal vein obstruction Budd–Chiari syndrome Chronic congestive heart failure
Malignancy		Leukaemia Hodgkin's disease Non-Hodgkin's lymphoma Metastatic disease Histiocytosis
Storage/infiltrative disorders		Lipidoses (e.g. Niemann–Pick syndrome, Gaucher's disease) Mucopolysaccharidoses (e.g. Hurler's syndrome, Hunter's syndrome) Amyloidosis Tangier's disease
Structural		Haematoma (trauma) Cysts or pseudocysts Haemangioma Lymphangioma

Table 7.5 Causes of massive splenomegaly (more than 8 cm below costal margin)

Infections	Parasitic	Chronic malaria (tropical splenomegaly) Schistosomiasis Visceral leishmaniasis (kala azar)
Extramedullary haematopoiesis	Haemolytic anaemia	Hereditary spherocytosis Thalassaemia major
Congestive	Portal hypertension	Non-cirrhotic portal fibrosis
Malignancy		Non-Hodgkin's lymphoma Metastatic disease Chronic myelogenous leukaemia (very rare)
Storage/ infiltrative disorders		Lipidoses (e.g. Niemann–Pick syndrome, Gaucher's disease)

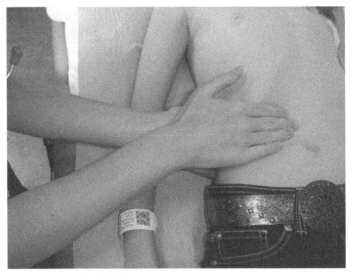

Figure 7.5 Bimanual palpation of right kidney.

percussed. Strike the dorsum of the middle phalanx by the tip of the middle finger of the other hand (the plexor) at 90°, with movement delivered from the wrist rather than the elbow. Once struck, lift the plexor immediately; the blow should be just hard enough to elicit the resonance.

Shifting dullness is useful for detecting moderate ascites and involves demonstration of a shift in the area of dullness with change of posture.

- Step 1: start in the centre of the abdomen to detect a resonant area due to gas in the bowel. If there is no area of resonance then the test cannot be performed. Move the pleximeter away from the resonant area and continue to percuss till you identify the upper border of the fluid in the midline (dull note).
- Step 2: place the pleximeter parallel to the flanks above the level of dullness and commence percussion. Continue to percuss and move slowly towards the flanks until a dull tone is elicited.
- Step 3: ask the child to turn to the side opposite to the dullness, while keeping the pleximeter at the site of dullness. After 15–20 seconds, repeat the percussion at the same site where dullness was elicited. If fluid is present, then the site will be resonant. Percussion away from this site will result in the return of a dull note. If there is no shift in area of resonance the presence of significant ascites is unlikely.

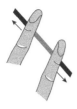 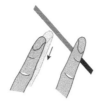 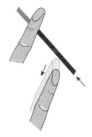

Step 1: Empty blood from the vein by placing two fingers on a segment of vein and moving them apart.

Step 2: Remove one finger and look for refilling of the vein. In this example the vein is not refilling.

Step 3: Replace the finger on the vein and then repeat step 2 but remove the other finger. In this example the vein has now filled up, indicating that blood flow is from below.

Figure 7.6 Determining the direction of venous blood flow.

Auscultation

Auscultation of the abdomen is performed to detect bowel sounds, rubs, and bruits. Warm the diaphragm of the stethoscope by rubbing with your hands. Apply it to the abdominal wall firmly but gently and auscultate various areas of the abdomen.

- **Normal bowel sounds** are heard irregularly every 5–10 seconds (but this can be up to a minute). Absent bowel sounds indicate paralytic ileus. Diarrhoea is associated with increased bowel sounds.
- **Bruit** is a blowing noise, which arises from stenosis of a large vessel such as the aorta or renal arteries, and is best heard with the bell of the stethoscope. Renal bruits are best heard over the renal angle or in the flanks (and can be easily missed by a nervous candidate!).
- A **venous hum** is usually heard over the right upper quadrant and is associated with enlargement of the anastomotic veins in portal hypertension. This sound is softer than the arterial bruit and tends to be continuous rather than systolic.
- **Rubs** are grating sounds caused by the rubbing of two inflamed and irregular surfaces against one another. They may occur over the liver, spleen, or an abdominal mass.

Examination of the posterior aspect of the abdomen

Inspection

As always start with inspection. The points to note are:

- asymmetry of the back
- spine:
  - contour: kyphosis, scoliosis, step-ups, prominent spinous process
  - skin: tuft of hair over the midline over the lumbo-sacral are may indicate spina bifida occulta
  - swellings: lipoma
- cutaneous haemorrhages: purpura, petechiae
- scars: midline scar (repair of neural tube defect, resection of spinal tumour), scars in the loin (nephrectomy, pyeloplasty)
- signs of inflammation: erythema, swelling, warmth, pain
- gluteal muscle wasting: sign of severe malnutrition
- perianal fissures and fistula: inflammatory bowel disease
- anus: patency, patulous anus may be seen in spina bifida.

Palpation

While examining the posterior aspect, the main objective of palpation is to identify any areas of tenderness. Tenderness could be present at one of the following sites: renal angle (pyelonephritis), bony prominence of the spine (tenderness may indicate infection, fracture, or malignancy) and paravertebral muscles (spasm).

Percussion

Percussion is mainly useful in identifying minimal tenderness over spinous processes. The plexor is tapped directly over the bony point without the use of pleximeter.

Auscultation

Auscultation is performed at the renal angles to look for the presence of renal bruit.

At the end of the examination, state that you would normally examine the genitalia and perform a rectal examination where indicated.

Other system examination

Other systems which may be examined depending upon the findings are cardiovascular, respiratory, and central nervous systems.

- cardiovascular system: pulmonary stenosis in Alagille's syndrome, patent ductus arteriosus in congenital rubella syndrome, dextrocardia in polysplenia/ asplenia syndrome
- respiratory system: cystic fibrosis
- central nervous system: hypotonia (Zellweger's syndrome), ataxia (vitamin E deficiency), chorea in Wilson's disease.

Common errors at this station

Common errors made by candidates that can result in failure of this station include:

- missing an enlarged organ such as a spleen or liver
- rough technique and causing pain to the child
- reporting physical signs that are not present
- poor examination technique
- failure to examine the back
- missing scars from previous surgery.

Videos

Video 7.1 In this station, Dr Zengeya examines the abdomen of an infant. This is a particularly difficult examination as the findings can be very easily missed. Note his gentle technique by which he ensures that the child does not get upset with the examination, and his identification of all relevant clinical findings.

Video 7.2 In this station, you can see Dr Zengeya assessing a mock candidate performing an abdominal examination. Notice that the candidate establishes good rapport and demonstrates his good technique while examining the abdomen. At the end, he summarizes his findings well.

Chapter 8 **Examination of the central nervous system**

Due to the complexity of the diseases and the number of tests involved, examination of the central nervous system (CNS) is relatively difficult in the exam setting. Candidates should realize that an attempt to carry out every aspect of the physical examination of the CNS will take too long and is obviously impractical. Appropriate signs need to be elicited quickly to identify the existence of a lesion, its anatomical localization, and likely pathology. Hence, the examination of this system requires plenty of practise and a polished technique. In the exam, you may be asked to examine, for example, just the motor system, or the upper or the lower limb, rather than an examination of the whole central nervous system. Prepare yourself for a screening examination, which will uncover most signs in a relatively short time. Remember, a detailed assessment of complex disorders is never a part of the MRCPCH Clinical Exam.

In this chapter, some areas have been explored extensively, keeping in mind the possibility of a 'small area' being examined. As the focus is mainly on examination technique and not theoretical aspects, basic neuroanatomy which has not been dealt with here should be read about elsewhere. Key competence skills required in the neurological examination are given in table 8.1.

Neurological assessment begins with the first contact with the child, that is the moment you enter the room. It is necessary to have a predetermined, systematic order of examination so that important signs are not overlooked. However, you should be ready to adapt the examination technique, depending on the child's age and the level of cooperation (e.g. compliant teenager, difficult toddler). Candidates should realize that a great deal can be learned by inspection before touching the child. Integration of observations with specific findings gathered during the neurological examination will fetch much credit.

Candidates are often not expected to reach a diagnosis in a short case. They are expected to define the deficit, decide on the anatomical level, if possible, and then consider the likely causes. Abnormalities commonly seen in the exam include cerebral palsy, hemiplegia, quadriplegia, diplegia, primary myopathy, and hereditary motor sensory neuropathies. It is productive to have a pattern recognition approach to neurological disorders. It is important to differentiate between upper motor neurone and lower motor neurone lesions. Upper motor neurone lesions present with universal weakness of muscles, more severe in the abductors and extensors in the upper limb and flexors and abductors in the lower limb, but with relatively normal muscle bulk.

Table 8.1 Key competence skills required in the neurological examination

Competence skill	Standard
Knowledge that the child is an individual and has rights	Demonstrate the ability to perform the physical examination with gentleness, respect, and compassion
Knowledge of descriptive terms of the nervous system	Demonstrate the ability to use the correct terminology for findings from examination of the nervous system
Knowledge and clear understanding of how to carry out a complete neurological examination	Demonstrate the ability to conduct a clinical examination in an organized fashion Examination of the motor system, including tone, power, and reflexes Sensory examination (superficial sensation, deep sensation, and cortical senses)
Knowledge of the systematic approach for examining the central nervous system	Demonstrate the ability to: identify an abnormality in the nervous system distinguish peripheral from central nervous system lesions
Summarize the findings, offer a differential diagnosis, and discuss a management plan	Demonstrate the ability to sum up the findings, provide the differential diagnosis, and offer an appropriate management plan

A complete neurological examination can be divided into seven areas:

1. general examination
2. assessment of the higher mental function including speech
3. cranial nerve examination
4. motor system examination (inspection, tone, power, reflexes, and function)
   a. upper limb
   b. lower limb
5. cerebellar examination
6. sensory system examination (pain, proprioception, vibration, touch, and higher sensory functions)
7. signs of meningeal irritation.

Tools required for the neurological examination are:

- reflex hammer
- 128 hertz tuning fork (for testing vibration and temperature sensation)
- ophthalmoscope
- visual acuity card (usually provided in the exam)
- a clean Q-tip.

General approach

These steps are repeated in every system to reiterate their importance and to help you recollect the initial approach of any clinical examination. Also refer to chapter 4.

- *On entering the examination room, adhere to infection control measures by washing your hands or using alcohol rub.*
- Introduce yourself *both* to the parents and the child.
- Ask the name and age of the child, if not already told by the examiner.
- Speak slowly and clearly with a smile on your face.
- Explain what the examination involves and obtain consent.
- Establish rapport with the child and parents.
- Expose the child adequately while ensuring their privacy. The child should be sufficiently undressed for the examination, but may need to be draped and a gown may be used to preserve modesty. Be careful with teenagers, who might resent being in minimal clothing. For examination of the upper limbs, expose both the upper limbs and the chest.
- Positioning: the child should be awake and alert, and the room should be warm and adequately lit. For assessment of the upper extremities, the older child may lie down or sit on the edge of the couch. It is preferable to examine the younger child on their parent's lap.

Visual survey—head to toe examination

The aim of the visual survey is to capture every available clue, which may help you to arrive at the correct diagnosis. Take a few seconds to watch the child actively at the start and continue to observe them attentively during the examination.

- Look at the child and try to estimate their approximate age.
- Always consider whether the findings combine to form a recognizable clinical syndrome. Common syndromes with motor involvement include Aicardi's syndrome, Angelman's syndrome, Arnold–Chiari malformation, Lesch–Nyhan syndrome, myasthenia gravis, neurofibromatosis,

Sturge–Weber syndrome, and Werdnig–Hoffman disease. Make sure you are familiar with common features of these conditions.

- Comment on the following:
  - ◆ state of wakefulness: awake/ aware/ alert/ active
  - ◆ general well-being: well, ill
  - ◆ attention, behaviour, interest in the surroundings, play, relation with parents
  - ◆ resting position
  - ◆ growth: comment on the nutritional status of the child; *comment that you would like to plot the child's height and weight on the growth chart.*
  - ◆ head:
    - ■ size: microcephaly/ macrocephaly
    - ■ shape: hydrocephalus, craniostenosis, small posterior fossa (cerebellar agenesis), occipital protuberance (Dandy–Walker malformation)
    - ■ sutures: separation, overriding, and fusion
    - ■ shunts and reservoirs
  - ◆ face:
    - ■ facial expression
    - ■ unusual facial features: facial asymmetry (VII nerve palsy), ptosis, dysmorphic facies (trisomy 21, fetal alcohol syndrome)
    - ■ eyes: squint, nystagmus, spectacles, Kayser–Fleisher rings of Wilson's disease
    - ■ secretions in the throat
  - ◆ skin: neurocutaneous markers, scars
  - ◆ degree of respiratory distress
  - ◆ tracheostomy scar
  - ◆ environment:
    - ■ wheelchair
    - ■ feeding pump, nasogastric tube (pseudobulbar palsy), feeding assistance devices such as PEG
    - ■ orthoses
    - ■ helmet
    - ■ spectacles
    - ■ ventilator
    - ■ urinary catheter
    - ■ dress
  - ◆ handedness:
    - ■ shake hand
    - ■ ask if right or left-handed.

Higher mental function

Examination of the higher mental function constitutes an integral part of the clinical evaluation of cortical function. A detailed assessment is time-consuming and not routinely performed. It is extremely unlikely that higher mental function will be assessed in the MRCPCH exam. For all practical purposes, one needs to have a simple instrument for screening cognitive dysfunction. Features of individual lobe lesions are given in table 8.2. In the section below, we have given modified mental assessment questions, which are suitable for children above 4 years. They concentrate on five areas of cognitive functions: registration, orientation, attention–concentration, recall, and speech (language) (acronym ROARS).

Table 8.2 Clinical features of cortical lobe lesions

Affected lobe	Clinical features
Frontal lobe	Changes of personality and behaviour (e.g. apathy or disinhibition)
	Loss of emotional responsiveness or emotional lability
	Cognitive impairments (particularly memory, attention, and concentration)
	Expressive dysphasia (dominant lobe)
	Conjugate gaze deviation to the side of the lesion
	Urinary incontinence
	Reappearance of primitive reflexes
Temporal lobe	Memory impairment
	Complex partial seizures
	Contralateral upper quadrantanopia
	Receptive dysphasia (dominant lobe)
	Anosmia
Parietal lobe	Signs of involvement of the dominant or non-dominant lobe
	Cortical sensory impairments (sensory and visual inattention, construction and dressing apraxia, spatial neglect and inattention, astereognosis, agraphesthèsia, tactile extinction, impaired two-point discrimination)
	Contralateral lower quadrantanopia
	Primitive reflexes
	Dysphasia (dominant)
	Signs of dominant lobe involvement
	Finger agnosia
	Acalculia
	Agraphia
	Left-right disorientation
Occipital lobe	Visual field defects (homonymous hemianopia)
	Visual agnosia (inability to read; word blindness)
	Visual hallucinations

- Registration:
  - Can you identify three objects by name?
- Orientation (person, place, and time):
  - What is your name?
  - Are you a boy or a girl?
  - Where do you live?
  - Where are you at the moment?
  - How old are you?
  - What time is it?
- Attention–concentration:
  - Can you count from 1 to 20?
  - Can you count backwards from 20 to 1?
- Recall (immediate):
  - Show the child three common objects and ask the child to recollect them.
- Speech (language):
  - Look at fluency and articulation of normal speech.
  - Name parts of the body.

- Simple command: Take the toy from my hand and put it on the table.
- Repeat a simple sentence (with a verb and a noun).
- Reading: Can you read your name?
- Writing: Write down your name.
- Copy a simple design.

Motor examination of the upper limb

Inspection

- **Posture**: note the resting posture. Look for abnormal flexion, unusual rotation or clawing of the hand. Always compare both sides for symmetry. In a child with hemiplegia, the upper limb is flexed at the shoulder and elbow with adduction and pronation of the arm, while the lower limb is extended.
- **Muscle bulk**: look for wasting (indicates denervation, myopathy, or disuse) and hypertrophy. Compare one side with the other and proximal with distal (asymmetry). Muscle wasting is not seen in acute upper motor neurone lesions.
- **Involuntary movements**:
  - fasciculation is fine irregular twitching of individual muscle bundles: ask the child to relax their arms and rest them on their lap; look at the large muscle groups for fasciculations; fasciculation, when present in association with weakness and wasting of muscle, indicates degeneration of the lower motor neurone
  - chorea is characterized by brief, jerky, irregular, quasipurposeful contractions that are not rhythmic
  - athetosis is characterized by continuous, slow, flowing, writhing, involuntary movements
  - dystonia is the slow development of an abnormal posture due to sudden, sustained contractions of the muscles
  - tics are sudden, repetitive, non-rhythmic, stereotyped motor movement or vocalization involving discrete muscle groups such as shrugging of shoulder
  - tremor is rhythmic, oscillatory movement across joints due to alternating muscle contraction and relaxation; look for tremors at rest while maintaining a posture and on active movement
  - myoclonic jerks are brief, involuntary, shock-like contractions of one or more groups of muscles.
- **Paucity of voluntary movements**
- **Contractures**
- **Scars.**

Palpation

For the rest of the examination, always explain the procedure to the child before carrying it out.

- **Tenderness**: ask the child 'Does it hurt anywhere?' This is to avoid manipulating any joint with tenderness.
- **Myotonia** (normal tone at rest, increased tone after active movement, and inability to relax the muscle): shake hands. If myotonia is present, the child cannot relax the handgrip and will open the hand slowly. This is seen in myotonic dystrophy.
- **Tone** (resistance felt when a joint is moved passively): in the upper limbs, tone is tested at the wrists and elbows. Ask the child to relax, let their shoulders and arms go floppy, and allow you to move the joints freely. Hold the child's hand below the wrists with one hand and support the elbow with your other hand. Flex, extend, and rotate the forearm at varying speeds. Assess the resistance to movements (both flexor and extensor tone) and decide if the tone is normal, decreased, or increased. Similarly, grasp the forearm proximal to the wrist with one hand and the child's hand with the other. Rotate the hand through the full range of movements, both slowly

and quickly. Hypertonia is present in upper motor neurone lesion (spasticity, which is velocity dependent resistance to passive movement) or extrapyramidal lesion (rigidity, which is sustained resistance throughout the range of movement). Rigidity is of two types, namely lead pipe and cogwheel rigidity (that is regular interruption to the resistance due to tremor). Hypotonia occurs in lower motor neurone lesion, cerebellar disease, early spinal shock, and in muscle disorders.

Power

- Assess muscle strength by comparing the child's strength against your ability to resist their voluntary movement.
- Start proximally and move distally. Compare both sides for symmetry.
- Demonstrate the movement to be performed to help the child understand.
- Palpate the muscle group as the child performs a movement.
- Assess the movements with gravity eliminated initially (direction of movement parallel to the ground), then against gravity, and finally against resistance.
- During routine assessment, quickly screen the proximal and distal muscle groups in each limb. If the power is reduced, then test the individual muscles.
- Determine whether the child has normal power by taking into account the maximum observed response and the age of the child.
- Grade the muscle strength using the Medical Research Council (MRC) scale (table 8.3).
- Shoulder:
  - Abduction—deltoid and supraspinatus (C5, C6): 'flex the elbow and abduct the arms'.
  - Adduction—pectoralis major and latissimus dorsi (C6, C7, C8): with the upper limbs abducted, ask the child to 'flex your elbows and pull your arms into your sides'.
  - Flexion—subscapularis and teres major (C5–C7): 'Bend your elbows and put your arms in front of your chest, as if to bear hug yourselves'.
  - Extension—latissimus dorsi and pectoralis major (C5, C6).
- Elbow:
  - Flexion—biceps, brachialis, and brachioradialis (C5, C6): 'Bend your elbow and do not let me straighten it'.
  - Extension—triceps and anconeus (C7, C8): 'Keep your elbow straight and do not let me bend it'.
- Wrist:
  - Flexion—flexor carpi ulnaris, and radialis (C6, C7): 'Bend your wrist and do not let me straighten it'.
  - Extension—extensor carpi radialis longus and brevis, extensor carpi ulnaris (C7): 'Stop me bending your wrist'.

Table 8.3 Medical Research Council scale for muscle power

Grade	Description
0	No muscle contraction
1	Flicker of contraction but no movement
2	Active movement with effect of gravity eliminated
3	Active movement against gravity but not against examiner's resistance
4	Active movement against gravity and resistance, weaker than normal
5	Normal power

- Fingers:
  - Flexion—flexor digitorum profundus and sublimis (C7, C8): 'Squeeze my fingers' or 'make a fist'.
  - Extension—extensor digitorum, extensor indicis, and extensor digiti minimi (C7, C8): 'Straighten your fingers and do not let me bend them'.
  - Abduction—dorsal interossei (C8, T1): 'Spread out your fingers and do not allow me to push them together'.
  - Adduction—palmar interossei (C8, T1): 'Hold your fingers together and stop me from spreading them out'.
- Thumb:
  - Extension—abductor pollicis brevis (C8, T1): Place the hand flat on the table with palm facing upwards and ask the child to 'Lift your thumb straight up to touch my pen'.
  - Opposition—opponens pollicis (C8, T1): Ask the child to 'Touch the tips of your thumb and little finger together' and try to break them apart.

Reflexes

- **Deep tendon reflexes** (contraction of a muscle elicited in response to sudden stretch of the tendon): the child should be relaxed and comfortable, as anxiety and pain can produce an exaggerated response. While delivering the blow, extend the wrists and allow the weight of the reflex hammer to deliver the impulse. Check the extent of the reflex contraction and the symmetry of the response. When a reflex is apparently absent, always test following reinforcement (isometric contraction of other muscles). In the case of upper limb reflexes, this can be done by asking the child to clench the teeth tightly just before the blow. Reflexes are graded according to the scale given in table 8.4. An abnormally brisk reflex (hyper-reflexia) occurs with upper motor neurone lesion. Diminished or absent reflex occurs with a lesion in the muscle, motor nerve, anterior horn cell, or sensory nerve.
  - **Biceps jerk (C5, C6)**: with the elbows semiflexed and forearm pronated, place the thumb on the biceps tendon, tap with the reflex hammer, and observe the arm movement. Normal response is a brisk contraction of the biceps with flexion of the forearm, followed by prompt relaxation. Repeat in the other arm and compare.
  - **Supinator jerk (C5, C6)**: with the elbows semiflexed and forearm semipronated, place the index and middle fingers on the lower end of the radius just above the wrist (styloid process) and then strike the fingers. Flexion of the elbow occurs as the normal response due to contraction of the brachioradialis.
  - **Triceps jerk (C7, C8)**: semiflex and support the elbow with one hand and tap over the triceps tendon. A normal response is triceps contraction, causing elbow extension.

Function

Assessment of function is useful in identifying dyspraxia (inability to perform a motor action despite understanding the task in the absence of motor weakness, coordination defects, or sensory impairment). To assess the functional capacity of the upper extremity, the following tests can be done

Table 8.4 Scale for grading the deep tendon reflex

4+	Very brisk, associated with clonus
3+	Brisker or increased than normal
2+	Normal
1+	Present but diminished
0	No response

- Give the child an object and see how they receive it.
- Ask the child to write on a piece of paper or draw a figure.
- Ask about 'combing your hair'.

Back examination

Motor examination of the upper limb is complete only after examining the upper back.

- Inspection: look for muscle wasting, winging of scapula, and surgical scars.
- Power (in addition to muscles of the shoulder, see above):
  - Serratus anterior (C5, C6, C7): 'Stand in front of the wall and push it with your hands'. Look at the back for winging of the lower scapula.
  - Infraspinatus (C5, C6): 'With your arms at your sides, bend both elbows to 90° and rotate the arms outwards (externally rotate)', while you provide the resistance against external rotation.

For features of individual nerve lesions, refer to table 8.5.

Motor examination of the lower limb

Inspection

Ask the child to lie down on the bed and expose to the underpants. Place a towel over the groin and inspect the lower limb.

- Posture: note the resting posture. Look for abnormal flexion or extension, unusual rotation, clawing of the foot, or limb shortening. Always compare with the other side for symmetry.
- Muscle bulk: look for muscle wasting of the quadriceps and anterior tibials, and hypertrophy of the calf muscles. Compare one side with the other and proximal with distal (asymmetry).
- Involuntary movements: look for abnormal motor activity such as fasciculations and tremor.
- Paucity of voluntary movements.
- Contractures.
- Scars, particularly on the posterior aspect of the lower limb.
- Equipment: urinary catheter, footwear.

Gait examination

Function assessment of the lower limbs is an important part of the neurological examination. Sometimes, this aspect alone is given as an individual case in the exam. It is important to remember that normal stance and gait depend on intact visual, proprioceptive, corticospinal, extrapyramidal, cerebellar pathways, and motor systems. There are two phases to the normal walking cycle: **stance phase**, when the foot is on the ground, and **swing phase**, when it is moving forward. While assessing gait, one should evaluate both the stance and walking, with various manoeuvres. Before the assessment, ask the child to remove their socks and footwear, and examine the shoe.

- Stance: make sure the legs and the thighs are clearly visible:
  - look for limb shortening
  - foot and knee position—valgus/ varus
  - width of stance
  - Romberg's sign (chapter 10).
- Walking:
  - Ask the child to walk normally, with a walking aid if needed, for a few metres and then turn around quickly and walk back. Look for age-appropriate walking, symmetry and smoothness of the gait, and ability to turn. Watch the width of gait, the arm swing and position, movement of

Table 8.5 Deficits in individual nerve lesions

Nerve	Motor supply	Motor deficit	Sensory deficit
Upper trunk of C5–C6 of brachial plexus (Erb's palsy)	Deltoid Biceps Brachialis	Loss of shoulder abduction, elbow flexion, and supination of the forearm Hand held in the waiter's tip position	Sensory loss over the lateral aspect of the arm and forearm
Lower trunk of C8–T1 of brachial plexus (Erb's palsy)	Intrinsic muscles of the hand Flexors of the wrist and fingers Dilators of the iris and levator palpebrae superioris	Claw hand with paralysis of all the intrinsic muscles ± Horner's syndrome	Sensory loss along the ulnar side of the hand and forearm
Radial nerve	Triceps Brachioradialis extensor muscles of the hand	Wrist drop Weakness of triceps when lesion is in upper third of the upper arm Loss of triceps jerk	Sensory loss over the dorsum of the hand and anatomical snuffbox
Median nerve (C6–T1)	Muscles of the anterior aspect of the forearm except flexor carpi ulnaris and the ulnar half of the flexor digitorum profundus Small muscles of the hand—flexor pollicis brevis, opponens pollicis, abductor pollicis brevis, lateral two lumbricals (FOAL)	Lesion at carpal tunnel: Weakness of abductor pollicis brevis and opponens pollicis Lesion in the cubital fossa: Ochsner's clasping test—ask the child to clasp the hands firmly together Inability to flex the index finger confirms a lesion on that side	Palmar aspect of the thumb, index, middle and lateral half of the ring fingers Palm is spared in median nerve lesions in the carpal tunnel
Ulnar nerve (C8–T1)	All the small muscles of the hand (except the FOAL muscles)	Wasting of the small muscles of the hand Clawing (hyperextension at the metacarpophalangeal joints and flexion of the interphalangeal joints) of the little and ring fingers Adduction of the fingers: place a card between the fingers and pull it out against resistance	Sensory loss on the palmar and dorsal aspects of the little finger and the medial half of the ring finger
Femoral nerve (L2, L3, L4)	Quadriceps Iliopsoas	Weakness of knee extension (quadriceps paralysis) Hip flexion weakness is only slight and adductor strength is preserved Absent knee jerk	Medial aspect of the thigh and leg
Sciatic nerve (L4, L5, S1, S2)	All the muscles below the knee Hamstrings	Foot drop Weakness of knee flexion Intact knee jerk but absent ankle jerk and plantar response	Posterior thigh, lateral and posterior aspect of the leg and the foot
Common peroneal nerve (L4, L5, S1)	Muscles of the anterior and lateral compartment of the leg	Foot drop Weakness of dorsiflexion and eversion of foot Intact ankle jerk	Minimal sensory loss over the lateral aspect of the dorsum of the foot

pelvis and knee, the heel lift, and toe push-off. Toddlers walk with wide, jerky steps. By age 7, children have a smooth, mature gait, with heel strike, stance phase (whole foot on the ground), push-off phase, and arm swing.

- ◆ Next, ask the child to 'walk heel to toe' in a straight line (tandem gait) to exclude a midline cerebellar lesion.
- ◆ Ask the child to 'walk on tiptoes' (to identify foot dorsiflexion weakness and S1 lesion).
- ◆ Ask the child to walk on their heels (a child with L4–5 lesion, foot drop, and Achilles' tendon contracture cannot do this manoeuvre).
- ◆ Ask the child to 'hop on each leg' (tests balance, coordination, and quadriceps function).
- ◆ Fog's test: 'walk on the outside (everted) of the feet'. This is useful in identifying mild hemiplegia and athetoid posturing of hands.
- ◆ Finally, ask the child to run (identifies subtle hemiplegia, which may be missed otherwise).
- • Other manoeuvres:
  - ◆ Gowers' sign: ask the child to squat and then stand up. This sign is present when the child uses the hands and arms to 'walk' up his or her own body from a squatting position due to weakness of the proximal muscles of the lower limb.
- • Types of gaits due to abnormal neurology (chapter 12):
  - ◆ Gluteus maximus gait: with weakness of the gluteus maximus, the trunk lurches backward at heel strike on the weakened side to interrupt the forward motion of the trunk.
  - ◆ Trendelenburg gait: during the stance phase on the weakened side, the pelvis tilts downwards to the opposite side. To compensate, the trunk lurches toward the weakened side (abductor lurch). This is seen in gluteus medius and adductor weakness.
  - ◆ Steppage gait: there is a difficulty in clearing the toes during the swing phase due to foot drop, therefore the child lifts the foot high off the ground to avoid tripping over and walks with exaggerated flexion at the knee and the hip.
  - ◆ Hemiplegic gait: the leg is extended at the knee and ankle and the foot is plantar flexed. The leg is swung in a lateral arc, with circumduction at the hip.
  - ◆ Scissors gait: flexion in the legs, hips, and pelvis with extreme adduction at the hips gives a crouched appearance. The knees and thighs cross each other while walking. This is seen in spastic diplegia.
  - ◆ Cerebellar gait: broad-based, unsteady, staggering gait, with a tendency to fall.
  - ◆ Toe walking: only the ball of the foot rests on the ground while the child is walking. Causes are spastic cerebral palsy, congenital short Achilles' tendon, and Duchenne's muscular dystrophy.
  - ◆ Waddling gait: broad-based gait with a duck-like waddle to the swing phase and tilt of the pelvis downwards to the side of the leg being raised and lumbar lordosis. It is seen in proximal myopathy.
  - ◆ Festinating gait: gait with stooped posture, short and shuffling steps, and loss of arm swing. It is seen in extrapyramidal disorders.

Palpation

Always explain the procedure to the child before performing it.

- • Tenderness: ask the child 'Does it hurt anywhere?' This is to avoid manipulating any joint with tenderness.
- • Tone: ask the child to lie down on their back. Assessment of the lower limb includes adductor tone at the hip, extensor tone at the knee, and plantar flexor tone at the ankle. A preliminary evaluation of tone can be done by rolling the legs from side to side. Next, place one hand under the knee and pull it up to check its tone. Then, support the thigh, and flex and extend the knee at varying speeds, while feeling for resistance (figure 8.1). Finally, check the tone at the ankle by plantar and dorsiflexing the foot, and assessing the resistance.

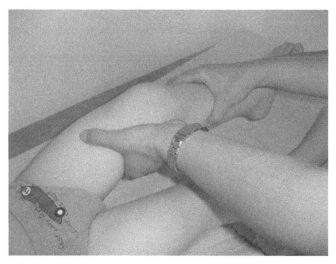

Figure 8.1 Testing for tone at the knee joint.

- Clonus: rhythmic contraction of the muscles evoked by sudden stretch. Ill-sustained clonus can occur in tired healthy individuals spontaneously, but sustained clonus indicates upper motor neurone damage. Clonus can be elicited at the knee and ankle.
  - ◆ Knee (patellar) clonus: with the knee extended, place the thumb and forefinger on the lower part of the quadriceps just above the patella. Push the patella down sharply towards the foot and sustain the pressure for a few seconds. In upper motor neurone lesion, sustained contraction of the quadriceps can occur while the downward stretch is maintained.
  - ◆ Ankle clonus: bend the knee and support the heel with one hand, sharply dorsiflex and partially evert the foot, and sustain the pressure for 2–3 seconds. When ankle clonus is present, rhythmical plantar flexion may occur until the dorsiflexion is sustained (figure 8.2).

Power

For general principles, refer to sections above.

- Hips:
  - ◆ Flexion—iliacus and psoas major (L2, L3): 'Lift your leg up and don't let me push it down' (place your hand above the knee).
  - ◆ Extension—gluteus maximus (L5, S1, S2): 'Push your heel down into the bed and don't let me pull it up'.
  - ◆ Abduction—gluteus medius, gluteus minimus, sartorius (L4, L5, S1): 'Spread your legs apart and don't let me push your knees together'.
  - ◆ Adduction—adductor longus, adductor brevis, adductor magnus, pectineus (L2, L3, L4): 'Keep your legs close together and don't let me push your knees apart'.
- Knee:
  - ◆ Flexion—semitendinosus, semimembranosus, biceps femoris, popliteus, gastrocnemius (L5, S1): 'Bend your knee and don't let me straighten it'.
  - ◆ Extension—quadriceps femoris (L3, L4): 'Bend your knee partially, straighten it and don't stop me from bending it'.

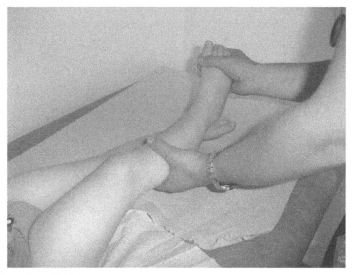

Figure 8.2 Testing for ankle clonus.

- Ankle:
  - Plantar flexion—gastrocnemius, soleus (S1, S2): 'Push the foot down and don't let me pull it up'.
  - Dorsiflexion—tibialis anterior, extensor digitorum longus, extensor hallucis longus (L4, L5): 'Lift your foot and don't let me push it down'.
  - Eversion (tarsal joint)—peroneus longus, peroneus brevis, extensor digitorum longus (L5, S1): 'Stop me turning your foot inwards'.
  - Inversion (tarsal joint —tibialis posterior, gastrocnemius, hallucis longus (L5, S1): 'Stop me turning your foot outwards'.
- Great toe:
  - Plantarflexion: 'Push the great toe down and don't let me pull it up'.
  - Dorsiflexion: 'Lift your great toe and don't let me push it down'.
- Reflexes.
- Deep tendon reflexes.
  - **Knee jerk (L3–4)**: ask the child to relax as much as possible. With the child lying on their back, slide one arm under the knees and lift to bend it slightly. Strike the infrapatellar portion of the quadriceps tendon directly with the reflex hammer. A normal response is the contraction of the quadriceps causing the knee to extend. Repeat on the other side and compare. At times, it might be difficult to elicit the knee and ankle reflexes, and a reinforcement manoeuvre should be used before deciding that reflexes are absent. The commonly used one is the Jendrassik's manoeuvre, which is performed by asking the child to interlock their fingers and pull the hooked fingers apart just before eliciting the reflex ('grip your fingers and pull your hands apart when I say "yes" ').
  - **Ankle jerk (S1–2)**: with the child lying on the back and fully relaxed, position the lower limb so that the thigh is externally rotated and the knee is partially flexed. Hold the foot in dorsiflexion with one hand. Strike the Achilles' tendon with the reflex hammer and note the plantar flexion. Compare both the ankle jerks.

- Superficial reflexes: contraction of the muscles elicited in response to light touch of skin.
  - **Abdominal reflexes** (above the umbilicus [T8, T9, T10] and below the umbilicus [T11, T12]): ask the child to lie down on the back and relax. With a blunt object, such as a key or tongue depressor, stroke briskly but lightly in each of the four quadrants of the abdomen in an inward direction, above and below the umbilicus. The normal response is the contraction of the underlying muscle with the deviation of the umbilicus outwards and upwards or downwards, depending upon the quadrant tested. Abdominal reflexes are absent in upper motor neurone lesions above the segmental level.
  - **Plantar (Babinski) reflex** (L5, S1, S2): ask the child to lie down on their back with legs out straight and relax. Using a blunt object, stroke the lateral aspect of the sole from the heel upwards and curve inwards across the ball of the foot medially. Stop before reaching the base of the great toe. In children older than 1 year, flexion of the big toe at the metatarsophalangeal joint is the normal response. The abnormal response, also called as positive Babinski's sign, is characterized by extension of the big toe and fanning of the other toes, and is seen in upper motor neurone lesion.
  - **Cremasteric reflex** (L1–2): this reflex is rarely elicited in the exam and is mentioned here only for the sake of completion. Ask the child to lie down on the back, abduct and externally rotate the thigh. With a blunt object, stroke the superior and medial aspect of the thigh in a downward direction. The normal response is the contraction of the cremaster muscle that pulls up the testicle on the side stimulated briskly.

Function

- Gait assessment—see above.

Sensory system examination

Detailed examination of the sensory system is time-consuming and difficult, and is rarely tested in the exam. In case you need to perform the sensory exam (e.g. child with sensory symptoms, spinal cord lesion, or peripheral nerve disorder), the following section will help you to cover the basics. The sensory exam includes testing for **superficial sensation** (pain, light touch, and temperature), **deep sensation** (proprioception and vibration), and **cortical senses** (stereognosia, graphesthesia, etc.). Nerve fibres carrying the pain and temperature impulses enter the spinal cord, crossover to the opposite spinothalamic tract after a few higher segments, and ascend to the brainstem. Proprioceptive fibres and touch fibres travel in the dorsal columns ipsilateral to the side of their origin until they reach the lower medulla, where they cross to the opposite side.

Children should be sufficiently undressed but draped to preserve modesty. Initial evaluation of the sensory system is done with the child lying on their back and eyes closed.

General principles

- Always test the sensation in a dermatomal distribution, proximal to distal, comparing the right with the corresponding area on the left. Move from an area of reduced sensation to normal or increased sensation. Map out the distribution of sensory loss and decide on the pattern of loss, which can conform to a region (spinal cord or upper brainstem lesion), dermatome (spinal cord or nerve root lesion), peripheral nerve, or glove and stocking distribution (peripheral neuropathy with involvement of multiple nerves).
- Often, in cases of spinal lesions, a level of increased sensitivity can occur above the sensory level, which usually indicates the highest affected spinal segment.
- Because the vertebral column is longer than the spinal cord in older children, spinal cord segments do not correspond to the vertebrae. The C8 spinal segment lies opposite to the C7 vertebra. The difference between the spinal segment and vertebra is about two segments in the upper

Table 8.6 Simplified dermatomal distribution

C4	Posterior aspect of the shoulders
C5	Shoulder tip and lateral aspect of the upper arm
C6	Lateral aspect of the forearm and tip of the thumb
C7	Tip of the middle finger
C8	Tip of the little finger
T1	Medial aspect of the upper arm and elbow
T4	Nipple level in the chest
T10	Umbilicus
L2	Upper anterior thigh
L3	Knee
L4	Medial aspect of the leg
L5	Lateral aspect of the leg and the medial side of the dorsum of the foot
S1	Heel and the sole
S2	Posterior aspect of the thigh
S3	Medial side of the buttock

thorax and three in the midthorax. Lumbar and sacral segments are found between vertebral levels T10–T11 and T12–L2, respectively.
- For a rough dermatome guide, refer to table 8.6 and figure 8.3.
- Always assess the cortical senses after establishing the intactness of the main senses and only when a parietal lesion is suspected.
- *Always explain the procedure to the child before performing it to decrease anxiety.*
- Avoid repetition of testing.

Superficial sensation (pain, light touch, and temperature)
- **Pain**: is almost never tested in the exam, unless it is absolutely necessary. Two types of pain sensation are tested during routine examination.
  - **Superficial pain**: with a new, disposable, neurological pin that does not penetrate the skin, touch a normal area and demonstrate the relatively sharp sensation with eyes open, to alleviate any fear of being hurt during the examination. Ask them 'does this feel sharp or blunt?'. Following this, ask the child to close their eyes and assess the pinprick sensation. Do not use a hypodermic needle.
  - **Deep pain**: squeeze the calf muscles or apply pressure to the nail bed. Ask the child to report when they feel discomfort.
- **Light touch**: following the principles of sensory examination discussed above, gently touch the skin with a cotton wisp in various places at irregular intervals. Ask the child to close their eyes and respond with a 'yes' every time they feel the sensation. Do not stroke the skin with the cotton wool.
- **Temperature**: ask the child to close their eyes, touch the skin with a cold tuning fork (which can be cooled by holding it under cold water) and ask 'Does it feel cold?'.

Deep sensation
- **Vibration**: *in contrast to spinothalamic senses, posterior column senses are tested from distal to proximal direction, as distal areas are the first ones to lose the sensation.* Strike a 128 Hz tuning fork

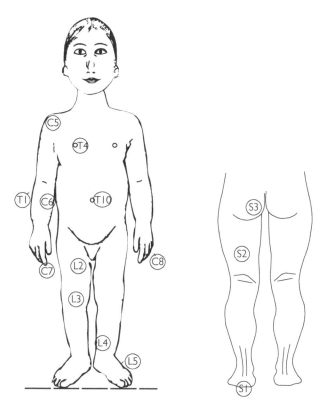

Figure 8.3 Simplified sensory distribution.

on your hand, place the handle of the vibrating tuning fork on the child's sternum and demonstrate. 'Can you feel the vibration (buzzing)? Tell me when it stops'. Test the vibration sense over the great toe, medial malleolus of the ankle, patella, knees and the anterior superior iliac spines in the lower limb and distal phalanx, styloid process of the radius, olecranon process in the elbow, and acromion process in the shoulder in the upper limb. Ask the child to close their eyes only if you are unsure about the response. There is no need to test the proximal areas if the sensation is perceived distally.

- **Proprioception** (joint position sense): hold the distal interphalangeal joint at the sides with the thumb and index finger of one hand and stabilize. With the child's eyes open, hold the digit distally from the side with the other hand, make small upward and downward movements, and finally hold it in one position, up or down. Then ask the child to 'tell me whether your finger is up or down'. Repeat the procedure with the eyes closed. Holding the top or bottom of the digit instead of the sides will produce pressure cues that will annul the test. Test the thumb and fingers in the upper limb and great toe in the lower limb, bilaterally.

Cortical senses

These are rarely tested in children and will not be discussed in detail here.

- **Two point discrimination**: ability to perceive two stimuli delivered close together as two different stimuli rather than one. The normal value over the tip of the fingers is 2–4 mm.

- **Graphesthesia**: ability to identify numbers or letters written on the skin with a blunt object.
- **Stereognosis**: ability to identify an object placed in the hand without looking at it.
- **Extinction**: ability to identify simultaneous stimuli delivered bilaterally to corresponding areas of the body.

Signs of meningeal irritation

Inflammation of the meninges leads to increased resistance to passive flexion of the neck and the extended leg. This can be identified clinically by eliciting neck stiffness, Kernig's sign, and Brudzinski's sign.

- **Neck stiffness**: with the child lying flat on their back, slip a hand under the occiput and gently flex the neck passively. In the presence of meningeal irritation, there is resistance to flexion of the neck due to spasm of the extensor neck muscles. Normally, the chin can be brought up to the chest wall.
- **Kernig's sign**: ask the child to lie down flat on the couch with both legs extended. Flex the hip and the knee to 90° on one side and then try to straighten the knee, while keeping the hip flexed. Kernig's test is positive when painful spasm of the hamstrings limits the extension of the knee, and at times the child will flex the head to avoid stretching of the meninges.
- **Brudzinski's sign**: ask the child to lie down flat on the couch with both legs extended. Flex the neck forward and look for flexion of the knees and hips.

Videos

Video 8.1 In this video Dr Chinthapalli demonstrates how to examine the upper limb. Notice how he quickly elicits the relevant clinical features of weakness and absence of reflexes. The examination is well structured, fluent, and is completed in the allotted time.

Chapter 9 **Examination of cranial nerves**

Cranial nerve examination is one of the commonly assessed areas of the nervous system in the MRCPCH clinical examination. The examiner may ask you to examine some of the cranial nerves or just the eye. This guide will take you through a systematic nerve examination, which is followed by most practitioners. You may need to individualize the examination sequence to suit your style. The key competence skills required in the cranial nerve examination are given in table 9.1. Cranial nerves cases commonly encountered in the MRCPCH Clinical Exam are listed in table 9.2. Causes of the different cranial nerve lesions are given in table 9.3.

General approach

These steps are repeated in every system to reiterate their importance and to help you recollect the initial approach of any clinical exam. Also refer to chapter 4.

- *On entering the examination room, demonstrate strict adherence to infection control measures by washing your hands or by decontaminating them with alcohol rub.*
- Introduce yourself *both* to the parents and the child.
- Talk slowly and clearly with a smile on your face.
- Establish rapport with the child and parents.
- Ensure privacy.
- Positioning: examine the older child while they sit on the edge of the bed or on a chair. It is preferable to examine the younger child on a parent's lap rather than on a couch, as this can cause much anxiety.

Visual survey—head to toe examination

The aim of the visual survey is to capture every available clue, which may help you to reach the correct diagnosis.

- Look at the child and try to estimate their approximate age.
- Always consider whether the findings combine to form a recognizable clinical syndrome. Common syndromes with cranial nerve involvement include Aicardi's syndrome, Angelman's syndrome,

Table 9.1 Key competence skills required in the cranial nerve examination

Competence skill	Standard
Knowledge of descriptive terms of the cranial nerves	Demonstrate ability to use the correct terminology for findings of the cranial nerve examination
Knowledge that the child is an individual and has rights	Demonstrates ability to perform a physical examination with gentleness, respect, and compassion
Knowledge and clear understanding of how to carry out a complete examination	Demonstrates ability to conduct a clinical examination in an organized fashion
Knowledge of the systematic approach to examining the cranial nerves	Demonstrates ability to examine all the cranial nerves
	Demonstrates ability to examine for motor strength
	Ability to assess various reflexes related to cranial nerves
	Sensory exam (touch, pain, vibration)
	Ability to assess special senses when appropriate (taste, smell, vision, hearing)
Summarize the findings, offer a differential diagnosis, and discuss a management plan	Demonstrate an ability to sum up the findings, provide possible differential diagnosis list, and offer an appropriate management plan

Table 9.2 Possible MRCPCH Clinical Exam cases with cranial nerve involvement

Cause	Diagnosis

Congenital	Moebius syndrome
	Syringobulbia
	Congenital intrauterine infections (CMV, toxoplasmosis, rubella)
	Congenital syndromes with:
	    visual loss
	    hearing loss: Pendred, Waardenburg, Treacher–Collins

Infective	Bell's palsy Guillain–Barré syndrome Postmeningitis, especially pneumococcal
Trauma	Head injury Horner's syndrome
Neoplastic	Brain stem astrocytoma Medulloblastoma

Table 9.3 Causes of cranial nerve lesions

Olfactory or cranial nerve I		Head trauma, damage to the ethmoid bone
		Frontal lobe tumour
		Foster–Kennedy syndrome (ipsilateral optic atrophy, central scotoma, anosmia, contralateral papilloedema)
		Kallmann's syndrome (hypogonadotropic hypogonadism with congenital anosmia)
		Refsum's disease (sensorimotor polyneuropathy, cataract, retinitis pigmentosa, anosmia, sensorineural deafness, and cerebellar ataxia)
		Idiopathic intracranial hypertension
Optic or cranial nerve II	Visual acuity (any abnormality of the lens, cornea, fundus, or optic nerve pathway)	Uveitis Cataract Lens dislocation Eye trauma Vitreous haemorrhage Optic atrophy Optic nerve hypoplasia Retinal detachment Retinopathy of prematurity Retinitis pigmentosa Stroke

	Visual field defects	Central field loss:
		    Optic neuropathy
		    Macular degeneration
		    Cone dystrophies
		Peripheral field loss:
		    Retinitis pigmentosa
		    Chorioretinitis
		    Glaucoma
		    Retinal detachment
		    Leber's optic atrophy
		    Hemianopia
		    Pituitary tumour
		    Optic tract lesion
		    Tumour in temporal, parietal, or occipital lobe
		    Migraine

Table 9.3 *Continued*

	Defective colour vision	Congenital colour vision deficiencies: Monochromacy Dichromacy Anomalous trichromacy Cone dystrophy Cone–rod dystrophy Achromatopsia Leber's congenital amaurosis Retinitis pigmentosa
Oculomotor or III cranial nerve	Pupillary abnormalities	
	Dilated fixed pupil	Internal ophthalmoplegia caused by a central or peripheral lesion Hutchinson pupil of transtentorial herniation Drugs Ocular trauma
	Adie's pupil	Viral encephalitis Familial dysautonomia (Riley–Day syndrome)
	Constricted pupil	Horner's syndrome Klumpke palsy Postcardiac surgery
	Nucleus, midbrain	Infarction Haemorrhage Abscess Malignancy
	Subarachnoid region	Meningitis Aneurysm Tumour and malignancy
	Cavernous sinus	Tumour and malignancy Aneurysm Arteriovenous fistula
	Eye	Hyperthyroidism Tumour
Trochlear or IV cranial nerve		Head injury Tumour Aneurysm
Trigeminal or V cranial nerve	Sensory	Herpes zoster Trigeminal neuralgia
	Motor	Bulbar palsy Myotonic dystrophy Poliomyelitis
Abducens or VI cranial nerve		Compression in the cavernous sinus, orbit, or base of the skull Aneurysm Head injury Increased intracranial pressure Meningitis
Facial or VII cranial	Congenital/ genetic	Myotonic dystrophy Moebius' syndrome Goldenhar's syndrome Osteopetrosis Trisomy 13 and 18

Table 9.3 *Continued*

	Trauma	Basal skull fracture Penetrating injury to middle ear Parotid surgery Birth trauma
	Neurological	Bell's palsy Guillain–Barré syndrome Myasthenia gravis Millard–Gubler syndrome
	Infection	Otitis media Herpes zoster (Ramsey–Hunt syndrome) Encephalitis Poliomyelitis Tetanus Lyme disease Botulism Diphtheria Cat scratch disease Acquired immunodeficiency syndrome
	Metabolic	Diabetes mellitus Hyperthyroidism
	Tumour/ malignancy	Leukaemia Metastatic carcinoma Neurofibromatosis
	Miscellaneous	Arsenic poisoning Cholesteatoma
Vestibulocochlear or VIII cranial nerve		Herpes zoster Neurofibroma Trauma Drugs (aminoglycosides, furosemide)
Glossopharyngeal or IX cranial nerve and vagus or X cranial nerve	Nucleus	Brain stem infarct Poliomyelitis Glioma Pseudobulbar palsy
	Base of the brain	Chronic meningitis Aneurysm Wegener's granulomatosis
	Peripheral	Perforating injury to the neck Diphtheria Botulism
Spinal accessory or XI cranial nerve		Trauma Cerebellopontine angle tumour Guillain–Barré syndrome Brainstem lesions
Hypoglossal or XII cranial nerve		Poliomyelitis Tuberculosis

Arnold–Chiari malformation, Crouzon's syndrome, Lesch–Nyhan syndrome, Sturge–Weber syndrome, and Werdnig–Hoffman disease.
- Comment on the following:
  - state of wakefulness: awake/ aware/ alert/ active
  - general well-being: well or ill
  - resting position
  - interest in the surroundings
  - growth: comment on the general nutritional status of the child but *mention that you would like to plot the child's height and weight on the appropriate growth chart*
  - head:
    - size: microcephaly or macrocephaly
    - shape: hydrocephalus, small posterior fossa (cerebellar agenesis), occipital protuberance (Dandy–Walker malformation)
    - sutures: separation, overriding, and fusion
    - shunts and reservoirs
  - face:
    - unusual facial features
    - eyes: squint, nystagmus, spectacles
  - neck:
    - tracheostomy scar
    - secretions in the throat
  - skin: neurocutaneous markers, scars
  - degree of respiratory distress
  - environment:
    - wheelchair: motor powered (indicates the child has sufficient intellectual ability and upper limb motor power to use the wheelchair) or manual (suggests the child has good upper body mobility or needs non-occupants to propel the chair)
    - feeding pump, nasogastric tube, percutaneous endoscopic gastrostomy (PEG)
    - orthoses
    - helmet
    - spectacles.

Individual cranial nerve examination

It is important not only to identify the cranial nerve lesion but also to classify its location as peripheral or central. Peripheral lesions are lesions of the cranial nerve or the nucleus, while central lesions are lesions of the brainstem, cerebrum, or cerebellum. An understanding of the functions of the cranial nerves is important and you need to study these from anatomy, physiology, or neurology textbooks.

Olfactory or cranial nerve I

The first nerve is not tested routinely, unless there is history of loss of smell (anosmia), head injury, signs of the frontal lobe lesion, or the examiner specifically seeks to do so. No localizing information can be gained from testing the olfactory nerve. When anosmia is present, the child often complains of altered taste. Pungent substances such as ammonia should not be used, as it is an irritant and the child can sense the noxious stimuli by sensory fibres of the trigeminal nerve. Common causes of anosmia are upper respiratory tract infection, congenital (Kallmann's syndrome), and post meningitis.

- First, note the external appearance of the nose. Then, examine the nasal vestibule by lifting the tip of the nose. Shut one nostril and ask the child to breathe through the other to check the patency of nasal passages.
- Once the patency is proven, ask the child to close their eyes and occlude one of the nostrils. Place samples of different substance with flavours familiar to the child such as coffee, soap, and peppermint near the nostril. Ask the child to identify the smell of the object. Make sure the stimulus is non-irritating, commonly used, and easily identifiable.
- Repeat the procedure to test the smell in each nostril separately.

Optic (ophthalmic) or cranial nerve II

Examination of the 'optic nerve' is different from examination of 'vision', as the latter involves assessing cranial nerves III, IV, and VI as well as cranial nerve II. In this section, we will concentrate on optic nerve examination, which is conducted under six subheadings: inspection, visual acuity, visual fields, pupils, colour vision, and fundus.

- **Inspection**:
  - Head position: if diplopia is present, the head is tilted to reduce double vision.
  - Eyelids:
    - Position, when looking straight ahead: ptosis (narrow palpebral fissure with the upper eyelid encroaching the pupil) can occur due to the lesion of the sympathetic pathway, which innervates the Muller's muscle, or the oculomotor nerve, which innervates the levator palpebrae. In myasthenia gravis, besides bilateral ptosis, one can notice wrinkled forehead, as the child reinforces eyelid opening with the frontalis muscle.
    - Lid lag: ask the child to look down slowly. Normally, the lid follows the downward movement of the eyes. In addition, see if the upper lid covers the sclera above the iris. Lid lag can occur in thyrotoxicosis, proptosis, or orbital mass.
    - Margin: look for inflammation.
  - Position of the eyeballs:
    - Proptosis: ask the child to sit on a chair, stand behind, and look down from above to see if the eyeballs protrude.
    - Enophthalmos: stand in front and look for obvious sinking by comparing one eye with the other. Bilateral enophthalmos is difficult to determine without radiographic studies or old photographs.
  - Periorbital area including the lacrimal apparatus: look for periorbital oedema, which is commonly seen in nephrotic syndrome, congestive cardiac failure, orbital cellulitis, and angio-oedema.
  - Conjunctiva: examine the lower lid by pulling it down with the thumb or index finger. Examine the upper lid by everting it, though this is not normally performed in the exam.
  - Sclera: comment on the colour (blue in osteogenesis and yellow in jaundice), and signs of inflammation.
  - Cornea: look for opacity, ulcer, and peripheral corneal deposition such as Kayser–Fleischer ring.
  - Iris: aniridia, heterochromia, Brushfield spots, etc.
- **Visual acuity**: any abnormality of the lens, cornea, fundus, or optic nerve pathway can reduce visual acuity. Assess both the uncorrected vision and vision corrected with spectacles, contact lenses, or a pinhole. Examine any child with uncorrected visual acuity of less than 20/20 with a pinhole. Improvement of vision through a pinhole indicates the error is refractive. In a toddler, visual acuity can be crudely assessed by using a toy. In children between 3 and 5 years, a Stycar matching letter test can be used. In older children, use a Snellen's chart or Logmar chart on the wall.

While testing one eye, cover the other. Test and record the visual acuity for each eye separately. Consider the possibility of an artificial eye, if the visual acuity is zero and pupillary reaction is not apparent.

* Check whether the child can count fingers held in front of each eye, perceive hand movements, or see light.
* If they can, then ask the child to sit 6 metres from the chart.
* Check to see if the child can read the top line and progressively smaller lines until they cannot go any further.
* If the child cannot read the top line at 6 metres, bring them forward to decrease the distance until they can see.
* Record the response as X/Y, where X is the line the child reads and Y is the line that a normal eye sees.

* **Visual fields**: the normal visual field extends to 60° nasally and superiorly, 100° temporally, and 75° inferiorly. The blind spot is located 15–20° to the temporal side of the point of visual fixation. In the clinical setting, visual field is tested by confrontation. While checking, some clinicians prefer to use white or red-tipped hatpin instead of wiggling fingers.
  * Remove the child's spectacles.
  * Sit facing the child with a gap of 1 metre, with your and the child's head at the same level.
  * First, perform a quick screening test of the major visual field defects. Keep your eyes open and ask the child to look at your nose. Wiggle the tip of your finger in superotemporal, superonasal, inferotemporal, and inferonasal quadrants. Ask the child to identify the moment when they see the moving finger.
  * Next, evaluate the visual fields by confrontation. Cover your left eye with your left hand. Request the child to cover their right eye with the right hand. Ask the child to focus on your left eye and say 'yes' when they can just see your wiggling fingers moving into sight.
  * Extend your right elbow and wrist to the side as far as possible, midway between yourself and the child. Wiggle the index and middle fingers and slowly bring them into the field of vision. Notice the point when your finger enters your field of vision and the point when the child sees the fingers, which should be similar. Continue moving the fingers until you reach the centre (to rule out any scotoma). Repeat this manoeuvre in each quadrant, and then with the other eye.
  * Finally, on the temporal field of each eye, continue to move the fingers horizontally across until it disappears from your visual field. Preserve the same temporal horizontal position, move it front or back until it disappears from the child's visual field. Map the blind spot and compare the size of the child's blind spot with yours. The blind spot is more accurately mapped using a red pin,

* **Pupillary examination:**
  * Resting appearance of pupils: ask the child to focus on a distant object, and note the size and symmetry of the pupils when the room is both dimly and brightly lit. Estimate the diameter of each pupil in millimetre. Unilateral mydriasis in bright light is seen in loss of ipsilateral parasympathetic innervation of the iris. Unilateral miosis in dim light is seen in ipsilateral sympathetic loss.
  * Light reflex: this comprises direct (constriction of the pupil of the stimulated eye) and consensual (constriction of the pupil of the unstimulated eye) reflexes. Place one hand vertically along the nose (to prevent focusing with both eyes and to avoid accommodation), and shine a light source from the side into one eye. Check for both direct and consensual response in each pupil on both sides. Presence of direct response in the right pupil without a consensual response in the left pupil suggests damage to the left oculomotor nerve or Edinger–Westphal nucleus of the brainstem. Absence of a direct reflex suggests total damage to the ipsilateral optic nerve.

- ◆ Swinging flashlight test: this is useful in detecting partial loss of sensory (afferent) stimulus to the brain. With a dim room light, ask the child to gaze into the distance and swing a light alternately from one pupil to the other. Observe the size and light reflexes of both pupils. Normally, both pupils constrict symmetrically, when one is exposed to light. When the light is shone on the eye with the afferent defect, both pupils will either constrict minimally or dilate. Light in the unaffected eye will cause a normal constriction of both pupils (Marcus–Gunn pupil).
- ◆ Accommodation: in a dimly lit room, ask the child to focus on the tip of your finger held about 1.5 metres away. Move the finger progressively closer to a point about 30 cm in front of the nose. Another method is to ask the child to look at a distant object and then at the tip of their nose. Look for convergence of the eye and constriction of the pupil. Accommodation is impaired in lesions of the optic pathway and oculomotor nerve. An intact accommodation reflex with absent light reflex can occur in Argyll–Robertson pupil (midbrain lesion) or Adie's pupil (ciliary ganglion lesion).
- **Colour vision**: colour vision is tested using Ishihara plates in older children. Ishihara plates consist of symbols made of coloured dots against a random background coloured spots. Defective colour vision is a sensitive test for optic neuritis. Impaired ability to identify red objects is an early indicator of optic nerve lesions.
  - ◆ Allow the child to wear their spectacles during the test.
  - ◆ Cover one eye and hold the plates about 35 cm from the face.
  - ◆ Ask the child to pick out the numbers written on the plates quickly.
  - ◆ Responses can be **anomalous** (colour-blind child gives different responses to colour-normal observers), **vanishing** (only the normal observer recognizes the coloured pattern), or **hidden** (only the colour-blind child sees the pattern).
  - ◆ Test colour vision of toddlers by asking them to identify various colours.
- **Fundus examination**: ophthalmoscopy involves not only fundus examination, but also visualizing the cornea, lens, vitreous, and choroids. Examine in a dimly lit room.
  - ◆ For proper fundus examination, the eye should be dilated using a mydriatic.
  - ◆ Examine the child with their spectacles in place.
  - ◆ Ask the child to keep still and fix their gaze on a distant target and to 'pretend' to see it, even if you obscure it with your head.
  - ◆ Approach the child from the side. For the right eye, hold the ophthalmoscope with your right hand and examine with your right eye to prevent the contact of your nose with that of the child. Keep your head vertical so that the child can fix with the left eye. Place your left hand on the child's forehead and gently retract the upper eyelid.
  - ◆ Remove your spectacles if you are a high myope or hypermetrope. Keep both eyes open, concentrate on the image from the right eye and suppress the one from the left eye.
  - ◆ Rotate the lenses clockwise to +10 diopter and observe the eye from 10 cm. Study the red reflex to detect any opacity (seen as dark patches against a red background) of the cornea, anterior chamber, or vitreous.
  - ◆ Slowly move closer to the child and simultaneously rotate the lens anticlockwise to reduce the power of the lens gradually. Focus will progressively shift from the lens, to the vitreous, and finally the fundus.
  - ◆ Once a blood vessel on the fundus has been located, follow it to locate the optic disc. Since the optic disc enters the eye nasally, approach the eye at a slight angle from the temporal side.
  - ◆ Observe the colour (normal—yellow, pale or white—optic atrophy), margins, and the cup of the optic disc and the pulsations of the optic vessels.
  - ◆ From the optic disc, follow the retinal blood vessels in four quadrants (superotemporal, inferotemporal, superonasal, inferonasal). The veins are large and dark red, while the arteries

are relatively thin and pale. Look for the presence of haemorrhages, microaneurysms, exudates, pigmentary changes, Roth's spot (suggestive of infective endocarditis), and white spots of choroiditis.

◆ Finally, with a smaller aperture beam, return to the disc, ask the child to look at the light and move nasally to view the macula along the visual axis.

Oculomotor (III), trochlear (IV), and abducens (VI) cranial nerves

Although each of these nerves control separate extraocular muscles, they are normally examined together due to their close functional interrelationships.

- **Inspection**: start with inspection of the eyes.
  - ◆ Head position: if diplopia is present, the head may be turned or tilted to minimize double vision.
  - ◆ Look at the eyelids and eye position.
  - ◆ Ask the child to look at an object about 1.5 metres away. Examine the size, shape, and symmetry of the pupils. Oculomotor nerve palsy causes mydriasis. Sympathetic palsy leads to miosis. Ciliary ganglion malfunction within the orbit produces Adie's pupil with mid-dilated pupils and poor response to convergence.
- **Ocular alignment**: the eyes are normally parallel in all positions of gaze except convergence. Squints can be either paralytic (paresis of one of the extraocular muscles) or non-paralytic (defective binocular vision). Congenital paralytic squints result in abnormal head postures, while the acquired ones cause diplopia. Non-paralytic (concomitant) squints are not associated with diplopia.
  - ◆ Looking at light: sit in front of the child about 1 metre away. Shine a light source and ask the child to look at the light. Observe the position of the light reflection on the cornea. Normally, the light reflex is symmetrical and slightly nasal to the centre of each pupil.
  - ◆ The cover test is a good test of eye alignment and is helpful to determine the presence of both manifest and latent strabismus.
    - Unilateral cover test: ask the child to focus on an object that is 3 metres away as if 'their eyes are glued to the object'. To test the right eye, cover the child's left eye with an opaque sheet and closely observe the movement of the right eye. Wait for 3–4 seconds to allow fixation of the eye. To test the left eye, cover the child's right eye and repeat the procedure. Absence of movement of either the right or left eye means the child does not have manifest strabismus. If the deviating eye moves inward after the other eye is covered, the child has exotropia (eye turns out). On the other hand, if the deviating eye moves outward, esotropia (eye turns in) is present (figure 9.1).
    - Alternating cover test: as before, ask the child to concentrate on an object that is 3 metres away. Cover the child's left eye with an opaque sheet for 1 to 2 seconds and then move quickly to the right eye. Hold the occluder in place for 1 to 2 seconds and repeat the cycle at least three times. As you unveil, observe the eye that is being uncovered to detect a refixation movement. Absence of movement means the child does not have latent strabismus. If the deviating eye moves inward after the other eye is covered, the child has exotropia. On the other hand, if the deviating eye moves outward, esotropia is present.
- **Ocular movements**:
  - ◆ Spontaneous movements of the eyes can be nystagmus or ocular bobbing.
    - Nystagmus is an involuntary rhythmic oscillation of the eyes in any direction (horizontal, vertical, or rotatory) and is characterized by a slow initiating phase and a quick corrective phase. The direction of nystagmus is defined by the direction of the quick corrective phase. To assess the nystagmus, ask the child to follow a fingertip held 30 cm away from the central gaze position to 30°. At times, nystagmus may be apparent only with gaze.

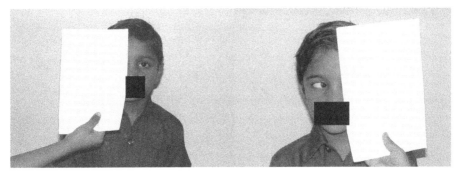

Figure 9.1 Unilateral cover test showing exotropia.

Jerky horizontal nystagmus may be caused by vestibular (direction away from the side of the lesion), cerebellar lesions (direction to the side of the lesion), and toxicity from alcohol or drugs such as phenytoin and benzodiazepines (both horizontal and vertical nystagmus). **Upbeat nystagmus** can be caused by lesions from the medulla to the midbrain, while **downbeat nystagmus** implies disorders of the craniocervical junction (Arnold– Chiari malformation). With **pendular nystagmus**, the velocity of oscillation is equal in all directions. It may be congenital or caused by either retinal lesions (decreased macular vision) or lesions of the central tegmental tract.

- Ocular bobbing is the abrupt, spontaneous, downward jerks of the eyes followed by slow drift to the midposition. It is characteristic of pontine dysfunction.

◆ Induced movements are used to assess failure of eye movement and diplopia. Sit in front, about 1 metre away and ask the child to follow your finger with their eyes while keeping their head still. Move your finger horizontally at the eye level, then vertically to the left at the lateral end (from the forehead to the chin), and, finally, to the right at the medial end, similar to a large 'H'. Look for lack of movement of the eyeball. Pause at the end of each direction to observe for nystagmus. Ask the child 'Do you see any double images (diplopia) in any direction' and if so 'when is it worse'. If diplopia is present, the false image is the one that is less distinct and more peripheral than the real one. The two images can lie side by side (horizontal diplopia) or one above the other (vertical diplopia). Cover one eye at the point when the diplopia is worst and find out which image disappears. Loss of the most peripheral image suggests the affected eye is the covered one. If diplopia persists after covering the eye, it indicates the presence of monocular diplopia, which can be due to astigmatism or a dislocated lens. Abnormal eye movement may be due to III, IV, or VI nerve palsy, gaze palsy, or internuclear ophthalmoplegia.

- III cranial nerve: in complete oculomotor nerve palsy, the affected eye will be in the down and out position, due to unopposed superior oblique (IV cranial nerve) and lateral rectus (VI nerve). The eye is incapable of movement upwards, downwards, or inwards. In addition, there will be ptosis (paralysis of levator palpebrae) and mydriasis. Only in partial oculomotor nerve palsy involving the inferior division is diplopia present, and it worsens on looking down and to the side of the lesion.

- IV cranial nerve: in trochlear nerve palsy, the child has either diplopia or head tilt. The child has compensatory head tilt away from the affected side towards the opposite shoulder to reduce their diplopia. Diplopia is best elicited when the child looks downwards and inwards, for example as if to read a book.

- VI cranial nerve: in abducens nerve palsy, the affected eye will have convergent squint. The child cannot move the eye past the midline outwards. Diplopia is maximal on looking to the affected side.

- Gaze palsy: this is the inability to move both eyes together in a single direction (horizontal or vertical) and can occur due to supranuclear (cortical gaze centres) or nuclear (brain stem gaze centres) lesions. In nuclear gaze palsy, the eyes can neither be moved voluntarily nor by reflex in the restricted direction. In supranuclear gaze palsy, only reflex movement is intact and voluntary movement is absent.
- Internuclear ophthalmoplegia: this is characterized by impaired adduction of the ipsilateral eye in horizontal gaze but not in convergence, due to an ipsilateral median longitudinal fasciculus lesion, which connects the sixth nerve nucleus, horizontal gaze centre, and contralateral third nerve nucleus. The resultant diplopia is worse on looking to the contralateral side.
- 'One-and-a-half' syndrome: this occurs because of a lesion affecting the horizontal gaze centre and the median longitudinal fasciculus on the same side. There is horizontal gaze palsy when looking to one side (the 'one') and impaired adduction on looking to the other side (the 'and-a-half') eyes. Convergence is unaffected.

Trigeminal or V nerve

The trigeminal nerve has three major branches: the ophthalmic nerve, the maxillary nerve, and the mandibular nerve. It is a mainly sensory nerve, but the mandibular nerve has a motor component to the muscles of mastication. Total loss of sensation in all three branches suggests the lesion is at the ganglion. A postganglionic lesion will result in total sensory loss in one division. Dissociated sensory loss (loss of pain and temperature sensation, but retention of touch) occurs with lesions of the medulla or upper spinal cord. Preserved pain sensation and lost touch sensation occurs with pontine nuclear lesion.

- **Sensory component**: proprioception is not tested on the face.
  - ◆ Sensation of face—touch:
    - Ask the child to close their eyes and say 'yes' when they feel the touch of an object on their face.
    - Touch lightly on the forehead (ophthalmic division), cheek (maxillary division), and next to the chin (mandibular division) on each side of the face with fingertip (gross touch) and then with a piece of cotton wool (fine touch). Do not stroke the skin, as it triggers pain and temperature nerves. Avoid the angle of the jaw, as it is innervated by the great auricular nerve.
    - Check if the strength of the sensation feels the same on both sides. If sensation is absent in an area, map the extent of the anaesthetic area.
  - ◆ Sensation of face— pain:
    - Show the disposable pin to the child and explain that you will touch with a sharp object. Reassure that it has not been used on anyone else. Demonstrate with their eyes open.
    - Ask the child to close their eyes.
    - Apply the disposable pin lightly in three different places (forehead for the ophthalmic division, cheek for the maxillary division, and next to the chin for the mandibular division) on each side of the face.
    - Ask if it feels 'sharp' or 'blunt', when you touch with the pin on their face. Compare both sides of the face.
  - ◆ Sensation of face—temperature:
    - Temperature it is not tested routinely, unless dissociated sensory loss is suspected.
    - To check temperature a tuning fork cooled by cold tap water can be used.
    - Follow the steps for examining the touch sensation, and check if the child can sense the chillness of the object.

- Corneal reflex: the afferent stimulus of the corneal reflex is carried by the nasociliary branch of the ophthalmic nerve and the efferent response is mediated by the facial nerve.
  - In the exam, omit the corneal reflex, unless there is sensory loss on the face or cranial nerve palsies.
  - Ask the child to look at a distant object, and approach from the side to avoid a visual threat.
  - Lightly touch the edge of the cornea (not the conjunctiva) with a wisp of cotton wool. Observe blinking of both eyes. Repeat the procedure on the other eye.
- **Motor component**:
  - Motor power: with a unilateral lesion, the jaw is pulled over to the paretic side by the pterygoids of the normal side. In unilateral upper motor neurone lesion, jaw opening and closing is normal due to bilateral innervation of both hemispheres to muscles that open and close the jaw.
    - Look for wasting of the muscles of mastication (temporalis, masseter).
    - Ask the child to clench the teeth. Palpate the temporalis and masseter, and feel the contraction as the child clenches the jaw.
    - Next, ask the child to open their mouth against resistance applied to the base of the chin, and note any deviation of the jaw (lateral pterygoids).
    - With their mouth open, ask the child to move the jaw from side to side against resistance (medical and lateral pterygoids).
    - Finally, ask the child to keep their mouth open and try to close the jaws with pressure on the chin (medial pterygoids).
  - Jaw jerk: this is normally absent, but is exaggerated in upper motor neurone lesion above the pons. Brisk jaw jerk by itself does not have any clinical significance.
    - Ask the child to let the jaw fall and open the mouth slightly.
    - Place your index finger on the chin and strike it with a reflex hammer gently to deliver a downward stroke.
    - Normally, the mouth closes slightly.

Facial or VII nerve

The motor fibres of the facial nerve supply the muscles of facial expression, the parasympathetic secretomotor fibres to the lacrimal, submandibular, and sublingual salivary glands, and the sensory taste fibres to the anterior two-thirds of the tongue via the chorda tympani. Clinical features of facial nerve palsy depend on the site of the lesion (table 9.4).

- **Inspection**: inspect the face during rest and while talking.
  - Facial asymmetry due to drooping of the corner of the mouth, smoothing of the wrinkled forehead, and the nasolabial fold and widening of the palpebral fissure. Asymmetry may not be seen in bilateral facial nerve palsy.
  - Spontaneous and involuntary movements of the face (hemifacial spasm orofacial dyskinesia, myokymia, or tics).
  - Lack of tears and dryness of the mouth.
- **Motor component**:
  - Demonstrate the actions and then ask the child to mimic.
  - Ask the child to do the following actions, look for asymmetry and check for the power of the muscles.
    - 'Raise your eyebrow and wrinkle your forehead' (frontalis).
    - 'Close your eyes tightly and stop me opening them' (orbicularis oculi).
    - 'Close your mouth and puff out your cheeks (orbicularis oris).
    - 'Show me your teeth' (buccinator) (compare the nasolabial grooves, which are smooth on the weak side).

Table 9.4 Clinical signs of facial nerve palsy depending on the level of lesion

Site	Manifestation	Explanation
Upper motor nerve (UMN) facial palsy		
Unilateral UMN (supranuclear) facial palsy	Weak muscles of the lower half of the face contralateral to the lesion with relative preservation of muscles of upper half	Part of the VII cranial nerve nucleus that supplies the upper face receives innervation from both cerebral hemispheres
Bilateral UMN (supranuclear) facial palsy	Loss of volitional movements of the face alone, preserved involuntary (emotional) movements	Due to the sparing of the extrapyramidal system which is responsible for the involuntary movements of the face
Lower motor nerve (LMN) facial palsy		
Unilateral LMN facial palsy at the nucleus	Ipsilateral weakness of all facial muscles with loss of both voluntary and involuntary movements of face	Loss of all the motor fibres to facial muscles
Unilateral LMN facial palsy at the cerebellopontine angle and in the facial canal between internal auditory meatus and nerve to stapedius muscle	Ipsilateral weakness of all facial muscles, loss of taste in the anterior two-thirds of tongue, hyperacusis, impairment of salivary and tear secretion	Loss of motor fibres to facial muscles, nerve to stapedius which dampens the ossicle movements and sensory taste fibres
Unilateral LMN facial palsy distal to nerve to stapedius muscle, but proximal to the stylomastoid foramen	Ipsilateral weakness of all facial muscles Loss of taste, impaired salivary secretion *No hyperacusis*	Loss of motor fibres to facial muscles Nerve to stapedius is preserved but sensory taste fibres are affected
Unilateral LMN facial palsy from the stylomastoid foramen	Ipsilateral weakness of regional facial muscles Preserved taste and salivary secretion	Loss of motor fibres related to site of lesion

- Bell's phenomenon: ask the child to close their eyes. In lower motor neurone VII nerve palsy, the upward movement of the eyeball is seen due to incomplete closure of the eyelid.
- **Taste sensation**:
  - Only in those with facial palsy, examine taste on the anterior two-thirds of the tongue.
  - Ask the child to protrude the tongue and not to speak during the test.
  - Apply a small sample of sugar, vinegar, salt, and quinine solutions (sweet, sour, salt, and bitter) with cotton buds to one side of the anterior two-thirds of the tongue, one at a time.
  - Ask the child to point to the taste on a prepared card.
  - Between each sample, rinse the mouth with water.
  - Repeat test on the other side of the tongue.

Vestibulocochlear or VIII cranial nerve

The vestibulocochlear nerve has two components, the cochlear branch provides innervation to the hearing apparatus and the vestibular branch is concerned with balance. Conduction deafness results from interference of sound wave transmission in the external canal or middle ear to the organ of Corti. In sensorineural hearing loss, the lesion can be in the inner ear, the vestibulocochlear nerve, or the brain. Because of the extensive bilateral connections of the ear, unilateral sensorineural hearing loss is usually due to the lesion of the nerve nucleus or the nerve itself. Bilateral hearing loss can be either due to a central lesion or bilateral exposure of the cochlear apparatus to toxins and infectious agents.

- **Auditory component**:
  - ◆ **Inspection**:
    - ▪ Remove hearing aids, while testing for hearing impairment.
    - ▪ Examine the pinna and look for scars behind the ears.
    - ▪ Do an otoscopic examination of both ears. Look for wax or other obstruction in the external auditory meatus and perforation of the tympanic membrane.
  - ◆ Whisper test: screening test for hearing loss in older children and correlates with a hearing loss of 30 decibels.
    - ▪ Stand about 1 metre behind the child on one side so that they cannot read your lips.
    - ▪ Close the external auditory meatus of the contralateral ear to mask the sound.
    - ▪ At the end of exhalation, whisper a word with two distinct syllables towards the ear that is being tested.
    - ▪ Ask the child to repeat the word.
    - ▪ Repeat the test on the opposite side.
  - ◆ Distraction test: this is a behavioural screening test of hearing for babies between 6 and 18 months. The test capitalizes on the infant's instinct to turn and locate a quiet sound presented at ear level outside the visual field.
    - ▪ In a quiet room, place the baby on the parent's lap, facing forwards.
    - ▪ Ask a helper (this could be your examiner) to stand in front of the child and capture his or her attention with a small toy.
    - ▪ Stand 1 m behind the child on a horizontal level at 45° outside the baby's field of vision.
    - ▪ Produce a sound stimulus with high frequency rattle.
    - ▪ See if the child turns and looks around for the source of the sound.
  - ◆ Weber's test: this test is for lateralization
    - ▪ Place the base of a vibrating 512 Hz tuning fork in the centre of the forehead.
    - ▪ Ask 'on which side the sound is louder'. Normally, it should be heard equally in both ears.
    - ▪ If sensorineural deafness is present, the sound is heard better in the normal ear. In conductive hearing loss, the sound is louder in the abnormal ear.
  - ◆ Rinne's test: this compares air conduction to bone conduction.
    - ▪ Place the base of a 512 Hz vibrating tuning fork on the mastoid process.
    - ▪ Ask the child to say 'now', when they can no longer hear the 'buzz'.
    - ▪ When the child indicates, remove the fork from the mastoid process and place the prongs of the tuning fork about 1 cm from the external auditory meatus.
    - ▪ Ask 'can you hear the sound now?' Normally, the sound is audible at the external meatus after it has disappeared from the mastoid process.
    - ▪ In sensorineural deafness, due to the universal decline of air and bone conduction, the note is audible at the external meatus similar to a normal child (Rinne positive).
    - ▪ In conductive hearing loss, bone conduction is better than air conduction and therefore, no note is audible at the external meatus (Rinne negative).
- **Vestibular component**: impaired vestibular function is one of the causes of difficulty in upholding posture, the others being defective proprioception and vision. To assess defective vision, refer to the optic nerve examination.
  - ◆ Vestibulospinal reflexes:
    - ▪ Romberg's test: stand close to the child to prevent them from falling over. Ask the child to stand upright with feet together, hands by the side, and eyes open. Note the balance.

Next, ask the child to close their eyes and observe them for a minute. In positive Romberg's test, the child sways or falls to the side of the labyrinthine lesion when the eyes are closed.
- Unterberger's stepping test: ask the child to walk on the spot (stationary stepping) with their eyes closed and arms outstretched for 30 seconds. In unilateral labyrinthine lesion, the body rotates to the side of the lesion.
- Nystagmus (see above):
  - Hallpike manoeuvre for positional nystagmus: ask the child to sit on the bed and turn their head to 45° on one side. Lay the child on the bed quickly with their head over the edge of the bed, 30° below the horizontal (support the head while the child lies down). Look for the presence and direction of the nystagmus. Repeat with the head turned to other side. This test is not normally performed in the exam.
  - Other tests of vestibular function, such as the oculocephalic and oculovestibular tests, are not performed in the exam setting and are not described here.

Glossopharyngeal (IX) and vagus (X) nerves

These two nerves are responsible for swallowing, phonation, and guttural and palatal articulation and are tested together in view of their close functional relationship.

- **History**:
  - difficulty in swallowing foods or choking
  - drooling of saliva.
- **Inspection**:
  - Ask the child to open their mouth and inspect the soft palate, uvula, and pharynx. Look for any displacement of the uvula and pooling of secretions.
  - Flash a light source into the mouth and ask the child to say 'aaah'. Look at the movements of the palate and uvula. Normally, the edge of the soft palate rises symmetrically and the uvula remains in the midline. In unilateral tenth nerve palsy, the edge of the soft palate does not rise on the affected side and the uvula is drawn towards the normal side.
- **Listen**:
  - Listen to the child's speech.
  - Note the quality and sound of the voice. Hoarseness of voice may occur with unilateral recurrent laryngeal nerve palsy (X nerve). Nasal voice may be seen in IX and X nerve palsy.
  - Ask the child to cough. Listen for the characteristic bovine cough, seen in recurrent laryngeal nerve palsy.
- **Motor component**:
  - Swallowing: ask the child to swallow a sip of water, and watch for any difficulty in swallowing, nasal regurgitation, or coughing.
  - Nasal air leak: ask the child to puff out their cheeks with the lips closed. Look and feel for air escaping from the nose. In IX and X nerve palsy, the soft palate does not rise and occlude the nasopharynx, resulting in air leak through the nose.
  - Gag reflex: do not test gag reflex in the exam.
- **Sensory component**: *testing pharyngeal sensation and the gag reflex are unpleasant for the child and should be omitted, unless there is dysarthria, dysphagia or lower cranial nerve palsies.*
  - Sensation: touch the posterior pharyngeal wall with a tongue depressor and ask if the child can feel the tongue depressor touching the palate. In IX nerve palsy, sensation is lost in the pharynx and posterior tongue.
  - Gag reflex: touch the posterior pharyngeal wall with a tongue depressor. Normally, there is reflex contraction of the soft palate and the child will gag. Intact sensation but absent gag suggests tenth nerve palsy. Do not test the gag reflex in the exam.

◆ Taste on the posterior third of the tongue: this is not routinely carried out. When performed, quinine should be used as the posterior third of the tongue is sensitive to bitter taste.

Spinal accessory or XI cranial nerve

The spinal accessory nerve is a motor nerve supplying the sternocleidomastoid and trapezius.

- **Inspection**:
  - ◆ Stand in front of the child and inspect the sternocleidomastoids for wasting or asymmetry. Palpate the muscles to assess their bulk.
  - ◆ Look from behind for wasting or asymmetry of the trapezius.
- Motor component: upper motor neurone lesion produces weakness of the ipsilateral sternomastoid and contralateral trapezius.
  - ◆ Trapezius: stand behind and ask the child to shrug their shoulders as hard as possible. Place your hands on the shoulders, and press down as the child lifts their shoulders.
  - ◆ Sternocleidomastoid: to test the left sternocleidomastoid, stand in front and ask the child to 'turn your head to the right against my hand'. Place your hand on the right side of the chin and resist the head turn. Repeat this procedure on the opposite side to test the right sternocleidomastoid. Normally, the child should be able to turn their head against resistance.

Hypoglossal or XII cranial nerve

The hypoglossal nerve provides motor supply to the intrinsic muscles of the tongue.

- **Inspection**:
  - ◆ Ask the child to open their mouth and inspect the tongue on the floor of the mouth. Observe the tongue for signs of wasting and fasciculations.
  - ◆ Next, ask the child to protrude their tongue. Look for deviation of the tongue from midline. In peripheral hypoglossal lesion, there will be atrophy and fasciculations, and the tongue will deviate towards the side of the lesion. In central lesion, there is spastic paralysis of the tongue without atrophy or muscle fibrillation and paralysis, and the tongue deviates to the opposite side.
- **Motor component**:
  - ◆ Ask the child to push their tongue into each cheek while you press from outside with your finger.

Videos

Video 9.1 In this station Dr O'Keeffe performs an examination of the cranial nerves on a young child. Notice his fluent systematic approach and his ability to turn this difficult exam into a game with the child. He summarizes his findings and offers a differential diagnosis.

Chapter 10 **Examination of the cerebellar system**

Although many books include cerebellar examination as part of the motor examination, it is discussed separately here in view of its importance. As children with cerebellar diseases are not often seen in routine clinical practice, candidates tend to neglect this system in their preparation and so find it difficult in the exam. Assessment involves examination of the gait and coordination, which tests both cerebellar midline and hemispheric function (tables 10.1 and 10.2). In the exam, you may pass through a station asking you to examine either the cerebellar system or the gait alone. If such an instruction is given, be clear what you need to focus on.

Key competence skills required in the cerebellar examination are given in table 10.3.

General approach

These steps are repeated for every system to reiterate their importance and to help you recollect the initial approach of any clinical examination. Also refer to chapter 4.

- *On entering the examination room, adhere to infection control measures by washing your hands or decontaminating with alcohol rub.*
- Introduce yourself *both* to the parents and the child.
- Ask the name and age of the child, if not already told by the examiner.

Table 10.1 Localization of cerebral lesions

Site	Location	Function	Clinical manifestation of lesion
Vermis	Midline of the cerebellum	Concerned with axial functions (posture, locomotion, position of head relative to trunk), control of voice and eye movements	Instability of the trunk and the legs while standing still or walking
			Dysmetric (wide-based compensatory) gait due to intention tremor of the legs
			Truncal imbalance—tendency to lean and fall toward the affected side in heel-to-toe tandem walking
			Retropulsion—strong tendency to fall backwards and the child appears to be actively pushing themselves backwards
			Ocular motor dysfunction—uncoordinated eye movements
Neocerebellum	Lateral cerebellar hemispheres	Planning of skilled voluntary movement of the ipsilateral limbs	Rhythmic intentional tremor (occurs on voluntary activity), worse when reaching for objects (finger-to-nose testing)
			Ataxia (incoordination)
			Dysmetria or past-pointing—overshoot or undershoot the target
			Difficulty in performing rapid repetitive movements—tapping fingers or feet
			Dysdiadochokinesis—difficulty in performing rapid, alternating movements such as pronation and supination of the hands
			Wide-based gait
			Excessive rebound—lack of checking movements
			Staccato speech—sounds drunken
			Hypotonia
			Pendular reflex
Flocculonodular lobe	Posteroinferior part of cerebellum	Vestibular functions and regulation of the vestibulo-ocular reflex	Nystagmus in different directions depending on which way the child is looking

Table 10.2 Cerebellar disorders in children

Chronic		
Congenital	CNS malformations	Cerebellar hypoplasia Vermian aplasia Dandy–Walker malformation Chiari malformation Joubert's syndrome
Hereditary	Autosomal recessive	Friedreich's ataxia Ataxia telangiectasia Abetalipoproteinaemia Vitamin E deficiency
	Autosomal dominant	Spinocerebellar ataxias
Acute/ subacute		
Infectious	Acute cerebellar ataxia Meningoencephalitis	
Immune-mediated	Acute disseminated encephalomyelitis Multiple sclerosis	
Drug/ toxin related	Alcohol Anticonvulsants Heavy metals	
Mass	Tumour Opsoclonus myoclonus syndrome (neuroblastoma) Arteriovenous malformation Abscess	
Trauma	Haemorrhage Vertebral artery dissection	
Miscellaneous	Basilar migraine Psychogenic gait disorder	

Table 10.3 Key competence skills required in the cerebellar examination

Competence skill	Standard
Awareness that the child is an individual with fully fledged human rights	Perform the physical examination with gentleness, respect, and compassion
Knowledge of descriptive terms of clinical findings relevant to the examination of the cerebellum	Demonstrate ability to use the correct terminology for the findings of the cerebellar examination
Knowledge and clear understanding of cerebellar functions	Demonstrate understanding that the cerebellum is important for coordination, equilibrium, and movements
Knowledge of the systematic approach to examination of the cerebellum	Demonstrates ability to examine specifically for coordination, tone, speech, and gait Demonstrates the ability to modify the clinical examination to suit the situation
Understanding that clinical features vary depending on the region of involvement	Demonstrate ability to localize lesions to the cerebellum based on clinical findings (see figure 10.1)
Summarize the findings, offer differential diagnosis, and discuss a management plan	Demonstrate ability to sum up the findings, to provide a possible differential diagnosis list, and offer an appropriate management plan

- Speak slowly and clearly with a smile on your face.
- Explain what the examination involves and obtain consent.
- Establish rapport with the child and parents.
- Expose adequately while ensuring their privacy.
- Positioning: to examine the older child, they may sit on the edge of the bed or on a chair when they are not acutely ill. It is preferable to examine the younger child on their parent's lap rather than on a couch, which can cause much apprehension.

Visual survey—head to toe examination

The aim of the visual survey is to capture every available clue, which should help you to arrive at the correct diagnosis.

- Look at the child and try to estimate the approximate age.
- Always consider whether the findings combine to form a recognizable clinical syndrome. Common syndromes with cerebellar involvement include ataxia telangiectasia, Dandy–Walker cyst, Chiari malformation, and Friedreich's ataxia.
- Comment on the following:
  - state of wakefulness: awake/ aware/ alert/ active
  - general well-being: well or ill
  - interest in the surroundings
  - resting position
  - growth: *comment on the general nutritional status of the child but mention that you would like to plot the child's height and weight on the appropriate growth chart.*
  - head and neck:
    - size: microcephaly/ macrocephaly
    - shape: hydrocephalus, craniostenosis (brachiocephaly, plagiocephaly, trigonocephaly), small posterior fossa (cerebellar agenesis), occipital protuberance (Dandy–Walker malformation)
    - sutures: separation, overriding, and fusion
    - shunts or reservoirs
    - unusual facial features
    - eyes: telangiectasia, squint, nystagmus, spectacles
    - tracheostomy scar
    - secretions in the throat
  - speech
  - skin: neurocutaneous markers, scars
  - degree of respiratory distress
  - environment:
    - wheelchair: manual or machine (independent use of a motor-powered wheelchair indicates the child has sufficient intellectual ability and upper limb motor power to use it)
    - feeding pump
    - orthoses: any devices used to support limb function
    - helmet
    - glasses.

System examination

While testing the cerebellar system, it is important to ascertain that the child has normal motor and sensory systems, as their lesions can result in abnormal tests of coordination, even without cerebellar lesions. If a child has difficulty in performing any of the tests for cerebellar function, separate assessments of power and proprioception should be carried out. Cerebellar signs should be tested only when the child has attained the appropriate developmental milestones in the respective areas (usually after 4–5 years).

As the spinocerebellar pathways are uncrossed, deficits from cerebellar damage are ipsilateral to the side of the lesion. In general, children with cerebellar lesions have postural instability, delayed initiation and termination of motor actions, inability to perform continuous, repetitive movements, and lack of smoothness and coordination of complex movements (figure 10.1). While examining, it is advisable to start from head to toe.

Head
- Look for **nystagmus**: involuntary, rapid oscillation of the eye in the horizontal, vertical, or rotatory directions, with the fast component maximal towards the side of the lesion.
- **Dysarthria** (staccato or scanning speech): listen to the child's spontaneous speech and watch for 'scanning speech' characterized by slow pronunciation and tendency to hesitate at the beginning of the word or syllable. It can be further tested by asking the child to say 'British constitution' or 'baby hippopotamus'. Look for poor modulation of the volume with irregular separation of syllables.

Upper limbs
- **Tremor**: look for resting tremor of the hands. Ask the child to pick an object and watch for intention tremor.
- **Hypotonia**: test the tone at the shoulders, elbows, and wrists. Ask the child to relax and not to resist. Move the limb at the joints passively at varying speeds, through several ranges of motion, and feel for lack of resistance or floppiness.
- **Dysmetria** (inability to perform point-to-point movements accurately) or **past-pointing**: for the finger-to-nose test place your index finger about 60 cm from the child's face. Ask the child to touch the tip of their nose with the index finger and then the tip of your outstretched finger with the same finger. Ask the child to repeat the movement as fast as possible while you slowly move your finger, ideally for 1 minute. Repeat the test with the other hand and compare. Normally, the child should be able to perform the movement accurately without overshooting or undershooting.

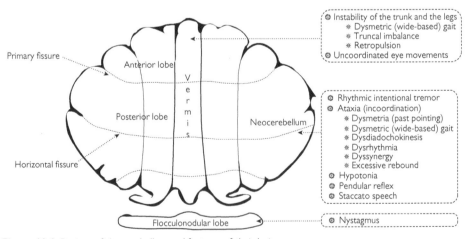

Figure 10.1 Regions of the cerebellum and features of their lesions.

- **Dysrhythmia** (inability to tap and keep a rhythm): ask the child to tap the table with the hand repeatedly or touch the tip of the index, middle, ring, and little fingers with the thumb rapidly to form circles with the fingers.
- **Dysdiadochokinesia** (inability to perform rapidly alternating movements): ask the child to place their hands on their thighs and then rapidly turn their hands over (pronation and supination of the forearm). Ask them to do this as fast as possible for 10 seconds and repeat the test with the other hand. A normal child should do so without difficulty.
- **Handwriting**: in children with cerebellar disorders, letters will be of unequal size, irregularly spaced, and the height of the letter increases while writing.
- **Rebound phenomenon**: place your left arm in front of the child's face for protection. Ask the child to flex their elbow while resisting the movement with your right hand. Release the resistance suddenly and look for inadequate braking of the forearm, which may fly upwards and may hit their face or shoulder (hence the need to use your left hand to prevent injury). Normally, the child can stop their arm in front of their face. *Remember that this manoeuvre is a recipe for disaster if it is not done well, as the child can injure themselves.*

Lower limbs

- **Gait** (refer to chapter 8): watch the different gait components (heel strike, toe lift off).
  - Step 1: ask the child to sit on the floor and then observe the child rising from the sitting position to rule out any proximal muscle weakness, which will prevent normal walking. Watch the stance while standing. Observe the posture and the steadiness of the child on their feet.

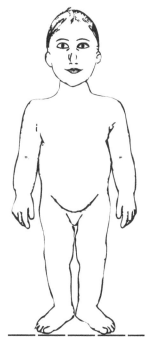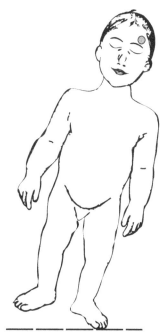

| Eyes open, arms by side and feet close together | When eyes closed, falls towards the side of the lesion |

Figure 10.2 Romberg's test.

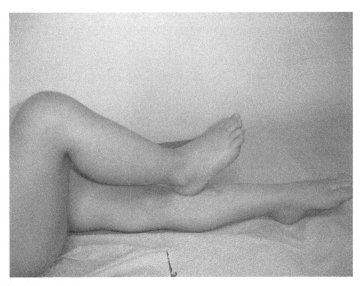

Figure 10.3 Heel-to-toe test.

- Step 2: ask the child to walk to the other side of the room and back. If the child normally uses a walking aid, observe the gait with and without it, if possible. Observe carefully for any gross gait abnormalities. Watch the walking base, the arm swing (a slight decrease is a sensitive indicator of upper extremity weakness), the heel lift, and toe push off. Note the turn around as this involves good balance and coordination.
- Step 3: instruct the child to walk in a straight line.
- Step 4: next, ask the child to walk heel to toe across the room (tandem gait) with their eyes open. Tandem walking should be possible without difficulty in children older than 4 years. A tendency to tilt or fall to one side indicates ipsilateral cerebellar lesion.
- **Romberg's test**: stand close to the child and be ready to support them in case of a fall during the test. Ask the child to stand unaided with feet together, arms by the side, and eyes open. Once the child is at ease in this position, instruct the child to close their eyes. If the child swings or loses balance, the test is positive (Romberg's positive). If they cannot balance with eyes open, do not ask them to close their eyes (figure 10.2).
- **Dysrhythmia, toe tapping**: to check for dysrhythmia (inability to repeat a rhythmic tap). Ask the child to perform rapid foot taps.
- **Postural stability (retropulsion)**: ask the child to stand with feet apart and eyes open. Explain that you will try to pull them back, but they must maintain stability and avoid moving backwards. Stand behind, close to the child, and be ready to catch them should they fall. Apply a quick pull backwards and look for an inability to maintain the stance. *This test is not performed routinely in the MRCPCH Clinical Exam.*
- **Pendular knee jerk**: ask the child to sit on the edge of the examination table with the legs hanging freely. With a reflex hammer, tap just below the patella. With cerebellar hypotonia, the leg swings freely (more than three cycles) like a pendulum, and eventually stop.
- **Heel-to-toe test**: finally, ask the child to lie down supine, place their heel on the opposite knee, and slide their heel down the shin to the top of the foot. Ask them to repeat the movement as quickly as possible a few times, before repeating the same with the other leg (figure 10.3).

Chapter 11 **Developmental examination**

All doctors working with children should have good knowledge of normal developmental milestones, as early diagnosis of developmental problems and appropriate intervention is desirable to improve the outcome. Candidates should be able to identify key warning signals and know the practical relevance of the milestones. 'Developmental assessment' is the comprehensive evaluation of a child's physical, intellectual, language, emotional, and social development, and is an area where most candidates lack competence and confidence. It should be distinguished from 'developmental screening', which is a brief, formal, standardized evaluation for the early identification of children at risk of a developmental disorder.

In the developmental assessment station, a candidate can be assessed in different ways: a developmental history with the parent and child; assessment of specific developmental domains (such as gross motor skills, fine motor skills, speech, language skills, etc.); or global assessment of an infant or older child. Occasionally, the candidate might be asked to just 'observe the child's play' and comment on the development. The candidate should anticipate and be prepared for these scenarios. In the exam, a detailed assessment of development is impossible, as it is complicated and time consuming. Ideally, observations of the child should take place with several people in varied settings, which is not feasible in the exam. However, useful assessment of a child's development can be easily performed as part of routine examination. The main purpose of the developmental assessment in the exam is to identify the child's strengths and weaknesses, the developmental problem, and, if possible, the cause of the problem. The candidate is expected to give an approximate developmental age at the end of the assessment.

Before we continue, it is important to understand the commonly used terminology. A child is said to have 'developmental delay' when he or she shows a significant lag (more than two standard deviations) in acquiring milestones in one or more domains. Global developmental delay is defined as a delay in two or more developmental domains. 'Developmental deviance' occurs when a child develops milestones outside or apparently ahead of the typical acquisition sequence. 'Developmental regression' is the loss of previously acquired milestones.

Children develop skills in various areas, also called developmental domains: gross motor, speech and language, fine motor, cognitive, personal–social, and emotional. For practical purposes, these domains are grouped into four: gross motor, language, fine motor – adaptive (including cognitive and fine motor) and personal–social (tables 11.1 and 11.2). It is essential to remember that there are large variations in normal development.

In this chapter, we aim to provide a basis for developmental history and structured developmental assessment. This chapter is divided into three sections: the first is on developmental history, the second is on developmental assessment of an infant, and the third is on developmental assessment of an older child.

Developmental history

The history is a major tool to gather information about a child's developmental achievements and parental concerns. It involves the comprehensive collection of information from parents or the caretaker on the progress of the child in all functional areas. A good developmental history uses the parent's valuable observational skills and elicits their observations, experiences, and concerns. High-quality information can be elicited by posing simple questions to the parents about the child's development.

For a productive developmental history, the establishment of rapport with both the parent and the child is the priority. All the techniques for establishing rapport that have been discussed in chapters 2 and 3 may be used for a successful interview. Observing the child's interaction and play during the interview can reveal a lot about the child's development and behaviour. It is important to engage the child during the encounter and encourage them to communicate. Here are some of the ways of keeping them engaged: discuss how they travelled to the hospital, their interests, hobbies, sports they follow, their toys, school friends, siblings, ambitions for the future, or recent events such as birthdays

Table 11.1 Developmental milestones in gross motor and psychosocial domains

Age		Eating	Dressing	Personal - Social		Gross motor
Range	Actual			Play	General/social	
0–3 months	6 weeks				Social smile	
	12 weeks				Recognizes mother	
4–6 months	16 weeks					Sustained head control
	5 months				Laughs	Rolls over supine to prone Reaches out for objects
	6 months					Transfers objects from one hand to another Rolls over prone to supine
7–9 months	7 months			Enjoys mirror	Stranger anxiety Prefers mother Responds to name	Sits briefly with support
	8 months				Object permanence Responds to 'No'	Crawl
	9 months	Chews biscuit		Plays peek-a-boo Plays pat-a-cake		Sitting without support Pulls to standing Creeps
10–12 months	10 months				Responds to words Waves bye-bye Will not give object to examiner	
	11 months				Looks for fallen object Will give object to examiner	Cruising
	12 months	Finger feeds		Simple ball game	Object recognition Releases object on request	Stands alone Walks with support

Age	Feeding	Dressing	Play	Social / Language	Gross motor
13–18 months 15 months	Picks up cup and drinks from it Uses cup and spoon			Indicates desire by pointing	Broad based gait Kneels Pushes wheeled toy
18–24 months 18 months	Feeds independently	Takes off socks and shoes	Symbolic play alone Dislikes being left alone Feeds doll	Points to named body parts Domestic mimicry Dry by day Obeys 2 simple orders Explores dustbins	Steady, purposeful walk Walks backwards Walks carrying toy Runs, squats Creeps downstairs
24 months	Feeds with fork and spoon		Role play Wants immediate satisfaction of needs	Toilet training Temper tantrums Obeys 4 simple orders	Walks up and down stairs holding on Kicks ball
30 months			Starts to play with other children	Dry by night Helps to put things away	Jumps Rises from knees without hands
25–36 months 36 months	Eats with fork and spoon ± knife	Helps in dressing	Vivid make-believe play	Likes hearing and telling stories Washes hands Brushes teeth Parallel play	Walks up stairs 1 foot and down 2 feet per step Stands on one leg Walks on tip-toes Throws ball Pedals tricycle
37–48 months 48 months		Able to undress	Dramatic make believe play Takes turns	Tells a story Goes to toilet alone	Walks up stairs & down 1 foot per step Hops
49–60 months 60 months	Uses knife and fork	Able to put on clothes and do up large buttons	Understands rules Chooses own friends Comforts playmate in distress		Skips Catches ball Runs on toes

Table 11.2 Developmental milestones in fine motor adaptive and language domains

Age		Vision	Fine motor	Hearing	Language
Range	Actual				
0–3 months	At birth	Follows a dangling ring at 25 cm 45°			Cry
	2 weeks			Startle responds to sounds	
	1 months	Fixate face and follows		Quietens, cries, or blinks to sound	
	6 weeks	Follows a dangling ring at 25 cm 90°			Vocalizes own sounds
	3 months	Follows a dangling ring at 25 cm 180°	Holds object for few seconds when placed in hands	Turns head at level of sound	Vocal play
4–6 months	4 months	Fixate on a toy brick	Reaches for objects without getting it Voluntary grasp		
	5 months		Reaches for objects and gets it		
	6 months	Adjusts position to see	Whole hand palmar grasp Mouthing Bidextrous approach Transfers from 1 hand to another	Turns head at below level of sound	Reduplicated sounds (Da, Ba, Ma)
7–9 months	7 months		Holds one brick when offered next		Makes noise for attention
	8 months			Formal Distraction Test	
	9 months	Looks at distant point when sitting	Grasps with finger and thumb, scissor fashion Throws toys to the ground Matching Index finger approach Finger thumb apposition		Variable babble
10–12 months	12 months		Good pincer grasp Casts repeatedly	Turns to name	2–3 words with meaning

Age range	Age	Vision	Manipulation	Counting	Speech/Language
13–18 months	15 months	Sees small objects	To and fro scribble Tower of 2 cubes Inserts pellet into bottle		Jargon speech 2–6 words Communicates wishes, obeys commands
18–24 months	18 months	Points to one object in picture card	Circular scribble Tower of 3 cubes Turns several pages of book Hand preference		6–20 words
	24 months		Copies vertical line Tower of 6 cubes Turns single pages of book		2 to 3-word sentences Uses pivotal grammar Uses questions
25–36 months	30 months		Copies circle Tower of 9 cubes		Refers self using pronoun 'I'
	36 months		Builds train and bridge if shown Draws a man with face and 2 other body parts		Gives first and last name Knows sex Recognizes 1 colour Lots of nursery rhymes
37–48 months	48 months		Copies cross Builds steps of bricks Draws a man with limbs and fingers	Counts 10 or more	Good account Enjoys long story Asks 'why' Recognizes 2 or 3 colours
49–60 months	60 months		Copies triangle Draws a man with recognizable face		Uses grammatical speech Asks 'when' and 'how' questions Enjoys joke

and festivals. Don't continue a conversation if the child is not interested in talking as this will waste valuable time. There is no standard developmental history checklist in children, however, a sample list is given in Box 11.1 at the end of this chapter. A developmental history should be adapted depending on the age of the child, the problems, and parental concerns. The developmental history should start from preconception and continue to the present. It should cover:

- the course of the pregnancy, complications, and details of recreational and therapeutic drug use
- the child's birth and neonatal period
- subsequent progress of the child's development in various domains
- protective factors as well as risk factors in children's lives.

Developmental assessment

Developmental assessment is the process of evaluating the maturity of the child by observing what the child can do and how they do it. In the examination, this can be in the form of clinical interview (see above), observation, or interaction with the child. The first method relies on a comparison of the milestones of the individual child to those of other children. The latter two methods depend on the child's 'performance' of certain tasks. A good assessment should incorporate all three methods so that it is valid and reliable. For assessment, tool kits containing items such as a rattle, crayons and paper, picture story book, doll, hairbrush, spoon, cup, bricks, and three or four piece of form board can be used. Most of these will be available in the examination room. However, it is useful and prudent to carry your own, familiar equipment.

The developmental examination is probably the most important station where the child's cooperation makes or breaks the case, therefore try to make 'friends' with the child. Get down to their level and avoid towering over the child. First, touch a non-threatening area, such as the hand, when handling a young child. Keep in mind that *observation* is the most important form of examination. Watching the child play can give a good overview of the developmental skills. It is equally important to talk to the child and the parents, while observing the social interactions. Remember to smile while talking to the child. Infants are best assessed with the parent next to them. In the case of toddlers and preschool children, initially make an informal examination while they are playing. Involve the parents to reassure the child and facilitate the examination.

General approach

These steps are repeated in every system to reiterate their importance and to help you recollect the initial approach of any clinical exam. Also refer to chapter 4.

- *On entering the examination room, adhere to infection control measures by washing your hands or decontaminating them with alcohol rub.*
- Listen carefully to the examiner's instructions (also known as the opening statement) and ask them to repeat if you are not sure.
- Introduce yourself *both* to the parents and the child.
- Ask the name and *age* of the child, if not already told by the examiner.
- Speak slowly and clearly with a smile on your face.
- Outline what you are going to do.
- Establish rapport with the child and parents.
- Ensure privacy.
- Positioning: the child should be awake and alert, and the room should be warm and adequately lit. Initial examination can be done on the parent's lap rather than on a couch separated from the parents. Later, after establishing rapport, the child can be encouraged to perform the manoeuvres without the parent at their side.

Box 11.1 Checklist for a child developmental history

Identifying information
Child's name
DOB/Age
How would you like me to call your child (any nick name) ?
Accompanying person and their relationship:
Contact details
General physician

Questions about the general health (be brief)
- List of major childhood illness, age of occurrence
- Hospitalizations, current medications, and allergies

Questions about developmental problems
- Do you have concerns about your child's development in any of the following areas? gross motor, language, fine motor–adaptive, and personal–social
- Please list any problems in the development of your child.
  - When did you first notice the problem?
  - What seems to make the problem better or worse?
  - Does your child have any special needs?
- Was your child specifically referred by someone? If so, whom?
- Has your child had previous assessments for the problem? If so, by whom and when?
- Has this child received any treatment? If so, please give the details of treatment (such as speech or occupational therapy and medication)

Pregnancy and birth
- Gestation?
- Mode of delivery?
- Child's weight at birth?
- Any complications during pregnancy, during, or immediately after delivery? If so, describe briefly

Milestones: at what age did this child do each of the following?
- Gross motor:
  - At what age did your child start to be able to hold their head still without support?
  - When did your child began to sit alone?
  - At what age did your child crawl? Was it 'all fours' crawling?
  - At what age did your child pull himself/herself up to chairs and tables?
  - At what age did your child walk with support and independently?
  - Does your child walk well without stumbling (when compared with peers)?
  - Does your child run a lot?
- Language:
  - What are the languages spoken in the home?
  - How well does your child speak the common language?
  - Any speech difficulties such as stuttering, stammering?
  - At what age did your child first make speech sounds?
  - When and what were the first words?
  - Age when your child said first sentences (combined two words).
  - Could people other than the family understand your child's speech?
  - Can the child understand other people.
  - Can the child say numbers from 1 to 10?
  - Knows how many fingers are on each hand.

- ◆ Compares things, for example, says 'this one is bigger, heavier,' etc.
- ◆ Counts three or more objects.
- ◆ Copies a circle or other shapes.
- ◆ Writes first name or part of it.
- Eating habits:
  - ◆ Age at which your child was weaned (bottle/breast).
  - ◆ Does your child eat with spoon, fork, hands?
  - ◆ Drinks from cup or bottle.
  - ◆ What hand does your child prefer to use for eating?
  - ◆ Is your child fed sitting in a high chair?
- Toilet habits:
  - ◆ Is your child toilet trained (day and night): 1. urination, 2. bowels?
  - ◆ Does child wear a nappy?
  - ◆ What is used at home? Potty chair? Special child seat? Regular seat?
  - ◆ Are bowel movements regular? How many per day?
- Dressing:
  - ◆ Can your child dress himself/herself?
  - ◆ Can they button clothes, zip zippers, lace shoes?
- Sleeping habits:
  - ◆ Does your child sleep in a cot or bed?
  - ◆ What time does child go to bed at night?
  - ◆ Are there any sleep time rituals?
- Play:
  - ◆ What are your child's favourite activities at home?
  - ◆ Where does your child usually play?
  - ◆ Is play active or quiet?
  - ◆ With whom does the child play—alone, siblings, peers, adults?
  - ◆ Does your child play well with other children?
  - ◆ Which foot is used for kicking?
  - ◆ Can he/she throw and catch a ball?
- Social behaviour:
  - ◆ Does your child get along well with adults?
  - ◆ Does your child get along well with other children (same age, younger, or older)?
  - ◆ Does your child like books and magazines?
  - ◆ Do you have any concerns about your child's behaviour?

Education
- Name of the school and their school year.
- How is your child doing at school?
- Does your child like school?
- Has the teacher reported anything about your child's schoolwork?
- Has your child ever repeated the school year? Why?

Family history
- Father's and mother's name, age, occupation, and consanguinity
- Siblings name, age, and sex
- What is the marital status of the parents—single, married, partnered, separated, divorced, widowed?
- Was the child adopted?
  - ◆ If yes, at what age?
  - ◆ What have you told your child about his/her adoption?
  - ◆ Does your child have any contact with birth parent(s)?

- Is there anything you would like us to be sensitive to about your child?
- Has any serious incidents/illnesses/changes occurred in your child's life recently?
- Are you getting any support from governmental agencies (for example, Sure Start)

Is there anything else we should know about your child?

- Comment on the following:
  - state of wakefulness: awake/aware/alert/active
  - general well-being: well, ill
  - attention, behaviour, interest in the surroundings, eye contact, play, relation with parents
  - concentration/distractibility
  - appearance: normal or syndromic
  - growth: whether the child is thin and small, thin and tall, well nourished and tall, well nourished and short. *Comment that you would like to plot the child's height, weight, and head circumference on the growth chart.*
  - head:
    - size: microcephaly/macrocephaly
    - shape: hydrocephalus, craniostenosis (brachiocephaly, plagiocephaly, trigonocephaly), small posterior fossa (cerebellar agenesis), occipital protuberance (Dandy–Walker malformation)
    - sutures: separation, overriding, and fusion
    - shunts or reservoirs
  - face:
    - facial expression
    - unusual facial features: facial asymmetry (VII nerve palsy), ptosis, dysmorphic facies (trisomy 21, fetal alcohol syndrome)
    - eyes: squint, nystagmus, spectacles, telangiectasia
    - secretions in the throat
  - posture
  - movements:
    - paucity of voluntary movements
    - presence of involuntary movements.

Developmental evaluation of an infant

As formal examination is difficult in infants, improvisation is often required. In general, it is better to start with non-threatening assessments such as vision, hearing, and language before proceeding to manoeuvres involving handling, such as gross motor assessment.

- **Vision**: babies with normal vision will fix and follow objects with their eyes. Dangle a ring at least 5 cm in diameter at 25 cm and move it in the horizontal plane. *Note the visual fixation and the ability to follow the ring.* A newborn can fix and follow up to 45°. At 6 weeks, the infant can follow up to 90° and up to 180° by 3 months. If the infant does not fix or follow the ring, look for the red reflex in each eye. In older children, check visual fixation with a brick or a Smarty. A baby can fixate on a 2-cm brick at 4 months, Smarties at 8 months, and distant objects at 9 months.
- **Hearing**: next, observe the response to sounds. Most crying babies will quieten to sounds by 1 month of age. *With the child sitting on the parent's lap, get down to the level of the ear and make a sound.* At 3 months, the infant turns their head to sound produced at the level of the ear. By 6 months, they turn their head to sound produced below the level of the ear. A formal

distraction test can be done at 8–9 months (see chapter 9). Although the startle response to loud noises is present in all babies with normal hearing, it should not be checked as it can cause significant distress to the baby.

- **Language**: once the normality of hearing is established, proceed to check the speech of the baby. *Listen to the sounds produced by the child and the response when you talk.* In the early stages of speech development, cooing (low soft and gentle cry, 3 months) and babbling (unintelligible sounds resembling language, 6 months) are heard. The baby learns to respond to their name by 8 months. Around 9 months, they begin to string sounds together, incorporate the different tones of speech, and say words such as 'mama' and 'dada' (without understanding the meaning of those words). They learn to say the first word with meaning at 1 year.

- **Fine motor–adaptive**: *Give a toy to the baby.* At 4 months, the baby reaches for it and by 5 months, they can reach and get the toy. Next, give a 2-cm brick to the baby. Look at the grasp, the ability to hold and retain, and to transfer to the other hand. A 6 month old holds the cube with the palmar grasp (curls the whole hand to wrap around the object) and 'mouths' the object. They can transfer the cube from one hand to another by 7 months. Give one more brick to the baby and observe the response. By 7 months, the baby holds on to both the cubes without dropping the first one. In older infants, give a pellet and look at the approach and grasp. At 9 months, the child reaches for the object with the index finger pointing at the object. They grasp the object between the thumb and radial fingers. At 10–12 months, the infant picks up a small object between the distal thumb and tip of the index finger. Check with the mother about finger feeding, which most can do by 1 year.

- **Personal–social**: *check with the mother about social smiling.* Social smiling occurs after 6 weeks in response to stimuli, such as talking or singing to the baby, and should be distinguished from spontaneous smiling, which occurs without any stimuli. The infant can laugh loudly at 5 months. Stranger anxiety (i.e. distress the child experiences when exposed to people unfamiliar to them) develops at 7 months, and can make the examination difficult. The infant can wave bye-bye at 10 months. *Give an object to the infant and ask him to give it back.* A child can do this at 11 months.

- **Gross motor**: testing for gross motor milestones should be kept for last. It is useful to follow the sequence of manoeuvres given here, starting with the supine position and moving on to the rest of the positions in a semicircle.

  - **Supine**: *observe the child while lying on the cot in the supine position.* Comment on the position of the head and limbs. A hypotonic baby will have extended limbs similar to a 'pithed frog'.
  - **Pull to sit**: *next, hold the baby by their hands and pull to the sitting position.* Look at the head lag and the ability of the baby to lift the head. By 4 months, head lag will disappear. At 5 months, the baby will lift the head in anticipation when about to be pulled up.
  - **Sitting**: *once the baby is pulled to the sitting position, look at the head control* (ability to support the head and sustain the position), *straightness of the back, and ability to sit independently without forward support of their arms.* Head control should be achieved by 4 months. An infant can sit with erect back at 6 months of age. Babies can sit with support by 7 months and without support by 8–9 months. They learn to pivot (rotate the trunk while sitting) by 11 months.
  - **Supported standing**: *place your hands in both axilla and lift the baby to standing position.* Look for weight bearing and standing. At 6 months, babies can bear most of their weight. At 36 weeks, they can stand holding on to furniture. At 11 months, they can cruise (walk holding on to furniture).
  - **Prone position**: *next, place the infant in the prone position. Look at the position of the head, arm, shoulders, and pelvis.* At 4 weeks, the head is turned to one side and the pelvis is higher than the shoulders. By 12 weeks, they can hold the chin and shoulders off the cot with the legs fully extended. By 6 months, they can hold the chest and upper abdomen off the cot, and can

role over from prone to supine position. They can crawl by 9 months, and creep on hands and knees by 10 months.

- ◆ **Ventral suspension**: *with your hands beneath the abdomen, lift the baby off the cot.* Look at the position of the head, limbs, and pelvis. At 6 weeks, the baby can lift their head to the horizontal plane momentarily; by 12 weeks, they can maintain the head above the plane of the body.

- **Primitive reflexes**: these are a set of transient reflexes which are evident in the neonatal and postneonatal period. They are called primitive because they are controlled by the most primitive parts of the brain, the medulla and midbrain. They are gradually inhibited by higher centres in the brain during the first 3 to 12 months of postnatal life. It is usually inappropriate to elicit primitive reflexes, unless you have noted asymmetry of movement of the limbs.

  - ◆ **Walking reflex**: this reflex is present from birth and disappears at 6 weeks. Hold the baby across the chest with your hands and allow their feet to touch the ground. The baby will try to make a 'walking motion' by placing one foot in front of the other.

  - ◆ **Moro's reflex**: this reflex is present from birth and disappears by 3 to 4 months of age. Hold the baby off the couch in the supine position with your arm underneath their back; lower the head and the upper back suddenly and unexpectedly by 'dropping' the baby a few inches. The baby will jerk up, throw the arms out, open the fingers with the palms up and then will bring the arms together while the hands clench into fists. At times, the baby might cry loudly. Asymmetrical Moro's is seen with a fractured clavicle and a brachial plexus injury.

  - ◆ **Tonic neck reflex**: there are two types—asymmetric and symmetric. The asymmetric tonic neck reflex is present from 1 month and disappears at 4 months. When the infant's head is rotated to the side, the arm on that side (face side) stretches into extension and the opposite arm flexes up above head (fencing posture). Persistence after 6 months would suggest cerebral palsy. The symmetrical tonic neck reflex is present from 4–6 months and disappears by 7–8 months. With the infant in the quadruped position on the floor, passively flex and then extend the infant's head. Flexion of the head causes flexion of the arms and extension of the legs, while extension results in extension of the arms and flexion of the legs. Persistence of this reflex will prevent the child from crawling.

  - ◆ **Galant's reflex**: this reflex is present from birth and disappears by 3–4 months of age. Hold the baby prone while supporting their belly with your hand and stroke the skin parallel to the spine. The infant will swing and flex the whole body towards the side that was stroked.

Developmental evaluation of toddler, preschool, and school-age children

In toddlers, the main domains of development are psychomotor and communication, whereas in preschool children most of the advances are in communication and language. In school-age children, social and behavioural aspects of development become more important. As the child gets older, gross motor milestones become less important (table 11.3).

- **Vision**: visual testing begins with assessment of visual acuity. The testing method varies, depending on age. Showing a colourful toy to toddlers and assessing their interest will provide a crude assessment of vision. In preschool children, vision (acuity and colour) can be assessed by presenting a series of simple pictures from a distance of 3 metres. For older children, vision can be tested using Snellen's charts (see chapter 9).

- **Hearing**: for hearing tests refer to chapter 9.

- **Language**: begin a conversation with the child; decide if the problems are receptive (impaired comprehension), expressive (impaired production), or a combination of both. At 1 year, the child can comprehend simple instructions and follow them. They can speak six or more words at 18 months. They can combine two words at 2 years, three words at 3 years, and four words at

Table 11.3 Developmental assessment of toddlers and preschool children

Communication by assessor	Expected response by the child
18 months	
Give simple instruction, e.g. 'give me the ball'	Follows the instructions
Talk to the baby	Says several single words
Show me your head, eyes, ears	Knows 2 or 3 body parts
2 years	
Show me, e.g. an object, a picture	Points to the object or picture
Show me body parts	Recognizes and shows body parts
Talk to the child	Uses simple phrases of two words
	Repeats words overheard in conversation
Give me, e.g. the ball and pen (two or more objects)	Gives as requested
3 years	
Show common objects and pictures	Recognizes and identifies almost all common objects and pictures
Talk to the child	Understands placement in space (on, in, under)
	Uses pronouns (I, you, me, we, they)
Ask their name, age, and sex	Tells the name, age, and sex
4 years	
Talk to the child	Speaks in sentences of 4 to 6 words
	Tells stories
5 years	
Talk to the child	Uses future tense
	Says name and address

4 years. In addition, the 3 year old can tell their name and sex, and use prepositions (in, on) appropriately. At 4 years, the child can follow a three-step command, count to four, name four colours, and enjoy rhymes. The 5 year old can count to 10 and respond to 'why' questions.

- **Fine motor–adaptive**: to test fine motor skills, you will need bricks, beads or pellets, book, pictures, paper, pencil, scissors, and form board.
  - ◆ **Bricks**: give a brick to the child and see the manner of grasp. Then ask the child to make a tower with the bricks. For smaller children, first demonstrate and then ask them to make the tower similar to what has been shown (figures 11.1 and 11.2).
  - ◆ **Beads or pellets**: next, place pellets on a flat surface, ask the child to pick them up and put them in a bottle. Look at the pincer grasp; a 15 month old can put the pellets in the bottle. At 18 months, the child can turn the bottle over and get the pellets out. For older children, give a bead and string and ask them to thread it, which a 3 year old can do.
  - ◆ **Books**: give a picture book and see how the child browses through the book. At 18 months, the child turns two pages at a time, while by 2 years, they can turn one page at a time.
  - ◆ **Pictures**: show the child a book of pictures and ask them to point out some common objects, which a 30 month old can do. Most children learn to identify colour by 4 years.

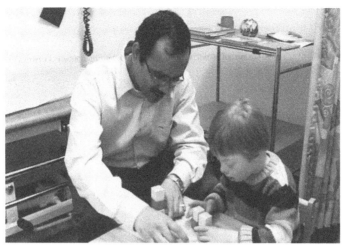

Figure 11.1 Assessment of fine motor skills using bricks.

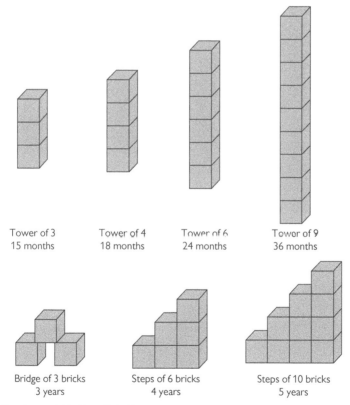

Tower of 3
15 months

Tower of 4
18 months

Tower of 6
24 months

Tower of 9
36 months

Bridge of 3 bricks
3 years

Steps of 6 bricks
4 years

Steps of 10 bricks
5 years

Figure 11.2 Developmental testing with bricks.

- **Paper and pencil**: you can ask the child to copy or draw geometrical shapes and draw a person or themselves (figure 11.3 and 11.4). The child's maturity is assessed based on the number of body parts in the drawing.
- **Paper and scissors**: a 3-year-old child can cut paper with scissors.
- **Form board**: ask the child to fill the shapes in a form board. The child can fit a circle and square at 18 months; circle, square, and triangle at 2–3 years, and six shapes at 4 years
- **Personal–social**: most of these milestones are based on history rather than examination.
  - **Feeding**: ask about drinking from a cup and feeding them self with spoon, fork, and knife. A 15 month old can drink from a cup and eat with a spoon without spilling. By 3 years, they are adept at eating with a fork and spoon; by 5 years, they can use a fork, spoon, and knife without difficulty.
  - **Dressing**: ask about dressing. At 14 months, the child starts helping to be dressed by putting their arms out. They help with putting shoes and socks by 18 months. By 3 years, children can dress and undress, except buttons and shoes, and can completely dress themselves by 5 years. They learn to brush their hair at 15 months.
  - **Self-care:**
    - **Toilet training**: most children are dry by day at 18 months and dry by night at 30 months
    - **Brushing teeth**: the majority of the children can brush their teeth by 3 years.
  - **Play**: children learn to play with dolls and brush the doll's hair at 18 months (figure 11.5). Children play next to each other, but do not try to influence one another's behaviour (parallel play) at 2 years. They learn to play with other children at 3 years and take turns while

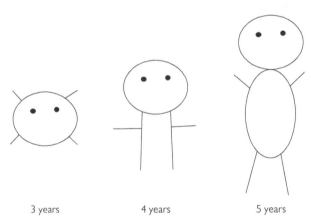

| 3 years | 4 years | 5 years |

Figure 11.3 Draw a person test.

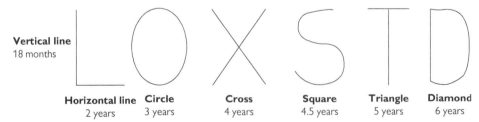

| **Vertical line** 18 months | **Horizontal line** 2 years | **Circle** 3 years | **Cross** 4 years | **Square** 4.5 years | **Triangle** 5 years | **Diamond** 6 years |

Figure 11.4 Geometrical shapes drawn at different ages.

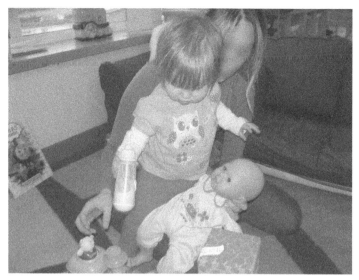

Figure 11.5 Playing with a doll at 21 months old.

playing at 4 years. By 5 years, they understand rules of a game and comforts playmate in distress.

- **Gross motor:**
  - ◆ **Locomotion**: while testing the locomotion, remember the following sequence—stand, walk, run, hop, and skip. Toddlers walk with a broad-based gait at 15 months. They can walk backwards at 18 months and run smoothly by 21 months. Preschool children learn to walk on tiptoe at 3 years. At the same age, they learn to stand on one leg and ride a tricycle. They can hop at 4 years and skip at 5 years.
  - ◆ **Throwing and kicking**: finally, give the child a ball and see them throw and kick. By 30 months, the child can throw and kick the ball and at 4 years, they are skilful at playing a ball game.

Videos

Video 11.1 In this station Dr Zengeya examines a mock candidate, Dr Dantuluri, performing a developmental assessment of the fine motor skills of a young boy. He uses appropriate tests and in the end gives a developmental age. He engages the child well. The candidate passed this station.

Chapter 12 **Examination of the musculoskeletal system**

The musculoskeletal examination, as for other systems, is best done in correlation with the medical history. You may be asked to examine the whole system, the spine, or a single joint. A structured approach is required, both for a screening examination and individual joint examination. Practise a systematic approach for presenting your findings, even if the examination is carried out in a different sequence from the one outlined here. Key competence skills required in the musculoskeletal examination are given in table 12.1. Musculoskeletal cases commonly encountered in the MRCPCH Clinical Exam are listed in table 12.2.

Stepwise examination of the musculoskeletal examination is performed as follows:

- visual survey (head to toe inspection)
- screening examination of the musculoskeletal system: gait, arms, legs, spine (pGALS)
- Examination of individual joints (hands and wrists, elbows, shoulders, head and neck, hips, knee, foot and ankle, spine):
  - ◆ look
  - ◆ feel
  - ◆ move
  - ◆ measurements
  - ◆ assessment of function
  - ◆ joint-specific tests.

General approach

These steps are repeated in every system to reiterate their importance and to help you recollect the initial approach of any clinical exam. Also refer to chapter 4.

- *On entering the examination room, demonstrate strict adherence to infection control measures by washing your hands or by using alcohol rub.*
- Introduce yourself *both* to the parents and the child.

Table12.1 Key competence skills required in the musculoskeletal examination

Competence skill	Standard
Knowledge of conditions with true joint and periarticular involvement	Ability to distinguish between true articular problems and conditions with periarticular involvement, which extend beyond the normal joint margin
Recognition of the involved structures and nature of pathology in musculoskeletal disorders	Ability to recognize joint, muscle and bone involvement in musculoskeletal disorders along with the pathology
Identify the extent and functional consequences of musculoskeletal disorders	Ability to perform screening exam of musculoskeletal system (pGALS)
Recognition of the effect of illnesses on the range of motion and function on various joints	Ability to perform a detailed musculoskeletal examination including the hip, knee, shoulder, hand, wrist, elbow, and back
Knowledge of the various paediatric musculoskeletal disorders	Ability to differentiate between normal and abnormal assessment findings Ability to produce a differential diagnosis of common musculoskeletal problems
Knowledge of systemic disorders affecting the musculoskeletal system	Ability to identify the presence of systemic or extra-articular manifestations in musculoskeletal disorders

Table 12.2 Musculoskeletal conditions that may be seen in the MRCPCH Clinical Exam

Primary cause	Disease	Musculoskeletal associations
Congenital	Skeletal dysplasias	Heterogeneous group, includes spondyloepiphyseal dysplasia, multiple epiphyseal dysplasia, achondroplasia
Infective conditions	Reactive arthritis	Painful, asymmetric oligoarthritis Often lower limb, enthesitis
	Tuberculosis	Ethnic background or travel Acute or chronic arthritis; spinal involvement
	Rheumatic fever	Painful, transient, fleeting arthritis
	Poststreptococcal reactive arthritis	Persistent, usually oligoarthritis
	Viral associated: parvovirus, EBV, CMV, rubella	Usually associated with fever, rash, oligo or polyarthritis, tenosynovitis
Autoimmune and inflammatory conditions	Systemic lupus erythematosus	Small joints of the hand and wrist usually affected, although all joints are at risk Remember blood pressure and urinalysis
	Juvenile idiopathic arthritis	Commonest chronic childhood inflammatory musculoskeletal condition Mild to severe Describe distribution of affected joint Signs of active disease Signs of damage and functional limitation Check eyes
	Juvenile dermatomyositis	Periorbital oedema, heliotrope discoloration, Gottron's papules, proximal muscle weakness Calcinosis and lipodystrophy in long-standing cases
	Scleroderma: localized or systemic	Tight, inelastic (hidebound) skin and subcutaneous tissue Raynaud's, digital pits, nailfold capillary changes, absorption of fingertips Underlying joint contractures Sometimes mimics juvenile idiopathic arthritis Localized form does not involve internal organs Systemic (rare) gut hypomotility, malabsorption and wasting, pulmonary fibrosis
	Henoch–Schonlein purpura Kawasaki's disease	Arthritis may be prominent
Hypermobility associated syndromes	Marfan's syndrome, Ehlers–Danlos, Down's syndrome, Larsen's syndrome, cutis laxa; osteogenesis imperfecta	Children can have pain from recurrent subclinical subluxation Most hypermobility is benign
Acute hip pain	All ages	Septic Arthritis or Osteomyelitis Can present as a limp, hip pain (radiates to groin), or knee pain
	0–3 years	Developmental dysplasia of hip
	3–10 years	Perthes osteochondritis of the femoral epiphysis
	10–15 years	Transient synovitis of hip Slipped upper femoral epiphysis
Secondary	Haemophilia	Acute haemarthrosis or chronic arthritis, often knee

- Talk slowly and clearly with a smile on your face.
- Establish rapport with the child and parents.
- Expose adequately while ensuring their privacy. Ideally, the child should be undressed to their underwear. If possible, watch the child undress.
- *Ask three important questions:*
  - Do you have pain anywhere?
  - Can you dress completely without difficulty?
  - Can you walk up and down the stairs without difficulty?
- Positioning: early in the examination, it is preferable to examine a younger child on their parent's lap rather than on a couch. Useful information can be obtained by watching the child walk and play. Depending on the joint, examine an older child either in the sitting or lying position.

Visual survey—head to toe examination

- Look at the child and try to estimate their approximate age, if not given.
- Always think whether the findings combine to form a recognizable clinical syndrome.
- Comment on the following:
  - state of wakefulness
  - general well-being
  - interest in the surroundings
  - size of the child
  - obvious lack of movement of a limb or joint
  - position and alignment of the spine and limbs
  - soft tissue: swelling, redness, muscle wasting, contractures, deformities
  - skin: scars, rashes, skin lesions
  - mouth, mucous membranes, teeth, and fauces
  - eyes: signs of previous iritis, lens dislocation, cataract
  - environment: splints, walking aids, or wheelchair.
- View the child in the **standard anatomical position** (standing with feet together, arms to the side and head, eyes, and palms of the hands facing forwards).
  - From the front:
    - bulk and symmetry of the shoulder
    - extension of the elbow
    - bulk and symmetry of the quadriceps
    - symmetry at the knee.
  - From the back:
    - alignment of the spine
    - bulk and symmetry of the gluteal muscles, hamstrings, and calf muscles
    - limb alignment
    - symmetry of the foot.
  - From the side:
    - cervical curvature
    - thoracic curvature
    - lumbar curvature
    - position of the knee
    - foot arches.

Screening examination of the musculoskeletal system

The movements tested below are the first to become affected if there is a problem with a joint or muscle. They are screening movements. Show the child the movement you want them to do, so that they can copy you. If any joint is painful or movement is restricted, then continue to the specific joint examination (modified from the pGALS screen).

Gait (walking)

There are two phases to the normal walking cycle: **stance phase**, when the foot is on the ground, and **swing phase**, when it is moving forward. The stance phase is further subdivided into the **contact** (outer border of the heel strikes the floor followed by pronation at the subtalar joint, which causes the tibia to rotate internally), **midstance** (loaded forefoot, supination of subtalar joint, which causes the tibia to rotate externally and the foot is converted to a rigid lever ready for propulsion), and **propulsive** (push-off) phases.

- Ask the child to walk normally with and without walking aids.
- Look for age-appropriate walking pattern: toddlers walk with wide jerky steps. By age 7, children should have a smooth, mature gait with contact, midstance (whole foot on the ground), propulsive phase, and arm swing.
- Look for symmetry and smoothness of the gait and ability to turn quickly.
- Ask the child to 'Walk on tiptoes/ walk on your heels'.
- Ask the child to 'Hop on each leg'. This tests balance, coordination, and quadriceps function.
- Types of gait:
  - Antalgic gait: shortened stance phase on the affected side. In addition, when the hip is the source of pain, there is lurching of the trunk towards the painful side during the stance phase.
  - Gluteus maximus gait: with weakness of gluteus maximus, the trunk lurches backward at heel strike on the weakened side to interrupt the forward motion of the trunk.
  - Trendelenburg gait: during the stance phase on the weakened side, the pelvis tilts downwards to the opposite side. To compensate, the trunk lurches toward the weakened side (abductor lurch). This is seen in gluteus medius and adductor weakness.
  - Steppage gait: there is difficulty in clearing the toes during the swing phase, due to foot drop. Hence, the child lifts their foot high off the ground to avoid tripping over and walks with exaggerated flexion at the knee and the hip.
  - Subtalar or heel pain: during the stance phase, the child avoids the heel strike and tenses the midfoot, in addition to a shortened stride.
  - Metatarsalgia: during the stance phase, the child avoids push off or walks on the side of the feet.
  - Toe walking: walks on the toes without putting much weight on the heel or any other part of the foot.
  - Trick movements: children with leg length imbalance swings the longer leg round and out to avoid tripping.

Arms

- General—ask the child to 'Put your arms out in front of you'. Look for:
  - muscle bulk
  - asymmetry
  - contractures and deformity
  - swollen joints
  - rashes (psoriatic, vasculitic, striae, Gottron's papules over knuckles)
  - scars.

- Hands:
  - ◆ Wrist or finger swelling and deformity: 'Put your hands out in front of you'.
  - ◆ Precision grip: 'Pinch your index finger and thumb together' and 'Touch the tips of your fingers with your thumb'. Children with involvement of the metacarpophalangeal joints will not do these movements.
  - ◆ Supination and pronation of forearm and flexion at the proximal and distal interphalangeal joint: 'Turn your hands over and make a fist'.
  - ◆ Extend wrists: 'Put your hands together palm-to-palm' (prayer position) (figure 12.1).
  - ◆ Flex wrists: 'Put your hands back-to-back'.
  - ◆ Look at the face and squeeze the metacarpophalangeal and other finger joints and wrist gently but firmly and ask if it hurts (tenderness indicates synovitis).
- Elbows:
  - ◆ Full extension: 'Arms out straight'.

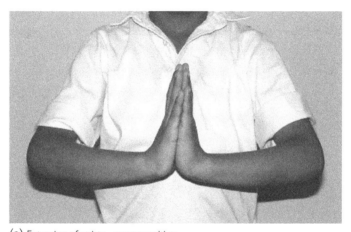

(a) Extension of wrists - prayer position

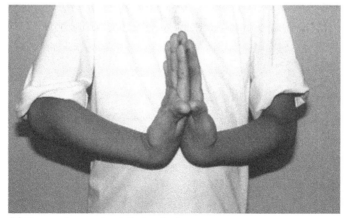

(b) Flexion of wrists - hands back to back

Figure 12.1 Flexion and extension at wrists. (a) Extension of wrists, prayer position. (b) Flexion of wrists, hands back to back.

- Shoulders:
  - ◆ Abduction: 'Reach up and touch the sky'.
  - ◆ External rotation of the shoulders: 'Bring your arms out to the side and put your hands behind your neck'.

Legs

- Hips:
  - ◆ Passively flex the knee to 90° and internally rotate at the hip (observe the difference between the sides).
  - ◆ In babies, examine the hip for dislocation and subluxation:
    - **Barlow's test** identifies an unstable hip that lies in reduced position but can be passively dislocated. Flex the hip and the knee, adduct the thigh, and push posteriorly in line with the shaft of the femur. In an unstable hip, the femoral head will dislocate posteriorly from the acetabulum, which can be felt as the femoral head slips out of the acetabulum (figure 12.2). Examine the hips one at a time.
    - **Ortolani's test** identifies a dislocated hip that can be reduced. Flex the hips and knees to 90°, abduct the thigh while placing anterior pressure on the greater trochanter using the index and middle finger. This brings the femoral head from its dislocated posterior position to the acetabulum and the hip reduces with a palpable and audible clunk (figure 12.3). Examine the hips one at a time.
- Knees:
  - ◆ Look for swelling or deformity of the knees and muscle wasting of the quadriceps.
  - ◆ Look for effusion at the knee (patellar tap).
  - ◆ Ask the child to bend and straighten the knee fully.

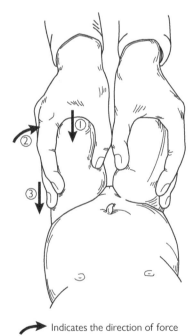

➤ Indicates the direction of force

Figure 12.2 Barlow's test. Arrows indicate the direction of force.

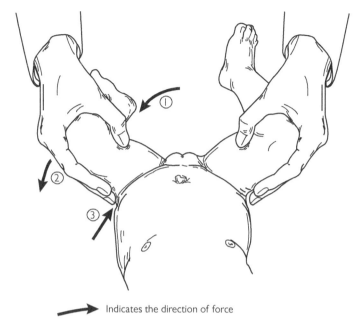

Indicates the direction of force

Figure 12.3 Ortolani's test. Arrows indicate the direction of force.

- Feet:
  - Look for callosities on the sole and arch of the feet and ankles.
  - Look at the face, squeeze the metatarsals gently but firmly side to side, and ask if it hurts (tenderness indicates synovitis of metatarsophalangeal joints).

Spine

- Inspection from behind:
  - look for
    - scoliosis
    - symmetry of the muscles
    - level of iliac crest
    - unequal buttock creases
    - keep the feet wide apart and check whether the lateral lumbar indentations 'dimples of Venus' are at the same level.
- Inspection from the front:
  - Lateral flexion at the neck 'Try to touch your shoulder with your ear'.
- Inspection from the side:
  - Look for normal curvatures: cervical lordosis, thoracic kyphosis, lumbar lordosis.
  - Forward flexion at lumbar spine and hip 'Can you bend and touch your toes, without bending your knees?'
  - Finger excursion for flexion: place two fingers on adjacent lumbar vertebrae. Your fingers should move apart as the child flexes forwards.
- Palpate down the spine and look for any signs of tenderness.
- Assess the degree of opening of the temporomandibular joint: 'Open your mouth and put in three fingers (i.e. child's fingers) sideways'. This is reduced in temporomandibular joint arthritis.

Detailed individual joint examination

When examining a specific joint, it is helpful to think in terms of: **look, feel, move, assess function, and joint-specific tests**. For the normal range of joint movements, refer to table 12.3. To determine the presence of hypermobility, calculate the Beighton score as given in table 12.4. *Before you start, ask the child 'Does anywhere hurt or is there pain at rest?'*

- Look (inspection):
  - ◆ Swelling: look for loss of normal contour and landmarks, distension, and fullness. Compare with the opposite side. To examine swelling around joints (synovitis, effusion) follow the shape of the joint capsule. To examine tendon swellings (tenosynovitis) follow the longitudinal line of the tendon sheath. Bony swellings are hard. Bursa are fluctuant and separate from the joint. Nodules are firm, subcutaneous, mobile, and often seen at sites of pressure. Calcinosis is hard and usually superficial.
  - ◆ Skin changes: redness.

Table 12.3 Range of motion of various joints in degrees (modified from JC Jacobs. *Pediatric rheumatology for the practitioner*, 2nd edn. New York, Springer, 1992)

Joint	Flexion	Extension	Internal rotation	External rotation	Abduction	Adduction
Neck tilt	45	50	80 (right)	80 (left)	40 (tilt)	40 (tilt)
TMJ	4 cm or 3 finger breadths (space between the incisors when mouth is fully open)					
MPCs	90	30–40		0		
1ˢᵗ MPC	70 (palmar)	09				
Wrist	80	70			20 (radial)	30 (ulnar)
Elbow	135	0–5	90 (supination)	90 (pronation)		
Shoulder	90	45	>55	>40–45	180	45
Hip	135	30	35	45	45–50	20–30
Knee	135	2–10			0	0
Ankle	50	20				
Subtalar			20 (inversion)	20 (eversion)		
Midtarsal					10 (midfoot)	20
1st MTP	45	70–90				

TMJ, temporomandibular joint; MPC, metacarpophalangeal joint; MTP, metatarsophalangeal joint.

Table 12.4 Beighton score for hypermobility

Passive little finger dorsiflexion beyond 90°	1 point for each hand
Thumb apposed to volar aspect of forearm	1 point for each thumb
Hyperextend elbow to >10°	1 point for each elbow
Hyperextend each knee to >10° (genu recurvatum)	1 point for each knee
Hands flat on floor without bending knees	1 point

Calculate total score. Hypermobile if score >4. Maximum 9 points.

- Alignment: angulation and deformity. Parents and children are sensitive to the word 'deformity'. Use terms such as malalignment, subluxation, dislocation, drift, or deviation.
- Changes to adjacent structures: muscle wasting.
- Feel (palpation):
  - Warmth: assess with fingertips for smaller joints and back of the hand for larger joints. Compare with an unaffected joint or the adjacent joint margins.
  - Tenderness: be careful and gentle if the area looks painful or tender. If the child complains about it in advance, do this as the last step. Squeeze a joint from the side until your finger and thumb just blanch. If you squeeze from above and below the joint, you may elicit pain from the tendon. Palpate the joint margin and adjacent bony structures and distinguish the tenderness from within and outside the joint.
  - Crepitus: coarse crepitus is produced from damaged joint surfaces while fine crepitus is usually from tendonitis.
- Move (active then passive) to examine:
  - Range of motion—compare both sides. Ask the child to show you what they can do with a joint themselves. For active movements, ask the child to move the joint through its complete range of motion and for passive movements, move the joints through the same range of motion with the child relaxed. Passive range of movements should be 5° more than active range of motion.
  - Pain during movements.
  - Stability: can the joint be moved into abnormal positions?
  - Muscle strength: ask the child to maintain a movement, while applying resistance on the opposite direction.
  - Assessment of function.
  - Joint-specific tests.

Hands and wrists

- Look:
  - Wrist or finger swelling and deformity: 'Put your hands out in front'.
  - Inspect hands (palms and backs) for joint symmetry, deformity, muscle wasting, palmar erythema rashes, and nail changes. Subtle hyperpigmentation over the knuckles may suggest early synovitis. Systemic lupus erythematosus rashes are seen between knuckles, while the rash in juvenile dermatomyositis is seen over the knuckles.
- Feel:
  - Assess skin temperature.
  - Bimanually palpate the wrists, metacarpophalangeal, proximal. and distal interphalangeal joints. Squeeze firmly and gently. *Watch the child's face for signs of pain*. Squeeze all joints laterally and not vertically. This distinguishes synovitis from tenosynovitis of the tendons.
- Move:
  - Assess the range of motion in the hand (active and passive):
    - Finger flexion and extension: 'Can you close and open the fingers of both hands?'
    - Precision grip: 'Pinch your index finger and thumb together' and 'Touch the tips of your fingers with your thumb'. Children with metacarpophalangeal joint involvement will not do these movements.
  - Assess the range of motion at the wrist:
    - Extend wrists: 'Put your hands together palm-to-palm' (prayer position) (Figure 12.1a).
    - Flex wrists: 'Put your hands back-to-back' (Figure 12.1b).
    - Supination and pronation of the forearm: 'Turn your hands over and make a fist' and 'Turn your palms up'.

- Squeeze the metacarpophalangeal and other finger joints and wrist gently but firmly. Look at the child's face and ask if it hurts (tenderness indicates synovitis).
- Assessment of function:
  - Ability to make fist.
- Joint-specific tests for carpal tunnel syndrome:
  - Tinel's sign: hyperextend the wrist and tap the median nerve with the middle finger or reflex hammer. The sign is positive if tapping elicits pain or paresthesias radiating down the palm in the index, middle, and outer half of ring finger (median nerve distribution).
  - Phalen's test: flex the wrist to 90° and maintain it for 1 minute. In a positive test, pain or paresthesias radiates along the index, middle, and outer half of ring finger of palm (median nerve distribution).
  - Carpal compression test: firmly compress the median nerve with your thumb at the flexor retinaculum, that is the carpal tunnel, for 30 seconds. A positive test producing pain or paresthesias in the median nerve distribution suggests median nerve compression.

Elbow

- Look:
  - Inspect for scars, swelling, or rashes.
  - Note any fixed flexion deformity.
- Feel:
  - Assess skin temperature.
  - Support the child's forearm, semiflex the elbow, and palpate the head of radius, joint line, olecranon process, medial and lateral epicondyles, and the extensor surface of the ulna. Tenderness of extensor tendons at the lateral epicondyle suggests tennis elbow.
- Move:
  - Assess active and passive movements.
  - Flexion and extension: 'Flex and extend your elbow'.
  - Pronation and supination: 'Keep your arms extended, supinate and pronate each hand'.
  - Note any hyperextension.
- Assessment of function:
  - 'Hand to nose or mouth'.

Shoulder

- Look:
  - Inspect the shoulder from the front, side, and behind for fullness, muscle wasting, and angulation. Shoulder effusions bulge anteriorly under the distal clavicle.
- Feel:
  - Assess skin temperature.
  - Palpation for tenderness: acromioclavicular joint for subacromial bursitis and intertubercular groove for biceps tendonitis.
- Move:
  - Assess (actively and passively) flexion, extension, abduction, adduction, external rotation, and internal rotation.
    - Flexion: 'Raise both arms forward and straight up overhead'.
    - Extension: 'Extend and stretch both arms backward behind your back'.
    - Abduction: 'With arms at your sides, lift both arms outwards and straight overhead'.
    - Adduction: 'Swing each arm across the front of the body'.

- External rotation: 'Place both arms behind your head, elbows out to the side'.
- Internal rotation: 'Place both the arms behind your hips, elbows out to the side'.
  - Ask the child to shrug their shoulders:
    - Observe the scapular movement, which should be symmetric.
  - Muscle strength testing
- Assessment of function
  - 'Keep your hands behind your head' and 'Put your hands behind your back'.
- Joint-specific tests:
  - Hawkins' impingement test: flex the shoulder and the elbow forward to 90° and internally rotate the arm. If this motion is painful, it is a positive sign for supraspinatus tendon impingement.
  - Neer's test: with the arm by the side of the trunk, elbow fully extended and internally rotated, and thumb touching the side of leg, forward flex the arm at the shoulder and move the arm up until it is above the head. Pain suggests impingement of posterior cuff.

Head and neck

- Look:
  - Look at the neck from the front, side, and behind for deformities and abnormal posture.
  - Assess the degree of opening of the temporomandibular joint: 'Open your mouth and put in three fingers (i.e. child's fingers) sideways'. This is reduced in temporomandibular joint arthritis.
- Feel:
  - Palpate the sternoclavicular and manubriosternal joints anteriorly and cervical spine, paravertebral, rhomboids, and trapezius muscles posteriorly for tenderness.
  - Place the index and middle finger of each hand in front of the tragus, ask the child to open and close the mouth and palpate the temporomandibular joint.
- Move:
  - Assess the active range of motion:
    - Flexion: 'Put your chin to your chest'.
    - Extension: 'Extend your head backwards'.
    - Lateral flexion: 'Touch your shoulder with your ear on the same side'.
    - Rotation: 'Turn your head and touch each shoulder with your chin'.
  - Joint-specific tests:
    - If crepitus is suspected in the temporomandibular joint, auscultate while the child opens and closes the mouth.

Hip

With the child lying on the couch:

- Look:
  - flexion deformity and leg length disparity
  - check for scars.
- Feel:
  - greater trochanter for tenderness.
- Move:
  - Assess flexion, extension, abduction, and adduction actively:
    - Flexion: 'Move your thigh up towards your tummy'.

- Extension: 'Lie down on your tummy, keep one leg straight, and lift the other leg off the bed without bending the knee'.
  - Abduction: 'Keep your legs straight (extended) and move your leg away from the midline'.
  - Adduction: 'Keep your legs straight (extended) and move your leg towards the midline and cross it'.
  - ◆ Assess flexion, extension, abduction, adduction, internal and external rotation passively.
    - Flexion: hold the heel and move the thigh up towards the trunk.
    - Extension: ask the child to turn to prone position, straighten one leg to stabilize the pelvis, and lift the other leg off the bed without bending the knee.
    - Internal rotation: flex the knee to 90° with the shin parallel to ground and the thigh in the perpendicular position, and move the ankle laterally.
    - External rotation: flex the knee to 90° with the shin parallel to the table and the thigh in perpendicular position, and move the ankle medially.
    - Abduction: with the knee extended, move the leg away from the midline.
    - Adduction: with the knee extended, move the leg towards the midline and cross it.
- Joint-specific tests:
  - ◆ Thomas' test: this is useful to detect occult hip flexion contracture. Flex the child's knee on one side and push firmly against the abdomen. The test is positive if the hip flexes and the thigh is off the table.
  - ◆ FABER test (flexion, abduction, external rotation of the hip) to distinguish hip or sacroiliac joint pathology from spinal problems: place the foot of the affected side on the opposite knee just above the patella (this flexes, abducts, and externally rotates the hip). Pain in the groin indicates a problem with the hip and not the spine. Gently, but firmly press the flexed knee and the opposite anterior superior iliac crest to the exam table. Tenderness in the sacroiliac area indicates a problem in the sacroiliac joints (figure 12.4). Repeat the manoeuvre with the other leg.
  - ◆ Straight leg raising test: with the lower limbs fully extended, lift the child's leg up to 70° from the table and then sharply dorsiflex the foot. The test is positive if pain increases in the lower back or leg. Pain in the leg produced from 0° to 30° indicates nerve root compression, between 30° and 60° suggests sacroiliac disease, and pain produced with leg motion beyond 60° points to lumbosacral conditions (figure 12.5).
  - ◆ Pelvic compression (to detect sacroiliac disease): with the child lying on the side, apply pressure to the hip joint. Repeat on the other side.
- Measurements:
  - ◆ Leg length: ask the child to lie down, make the pelvis 'square' (both anterior superior iliac spine at the same level) and measure from the anterior superior iliac spine to the medial malleolus.
  With the child standing:
- Look:
  - ◆ Gluteal muscle bulk.
- Move:
  - ◆ Assess the child's gait.
    - Mobility and gait: refer to the section on screening examination.
- Joint-specific tests:
  - ◆ Trendelenburg's test: ask the child to lift one leg. Watch for the tilt of the pelvis on the non-weight-bearing side. When positive, the pelvis tilts downwards instead of raising on the side of the lifted foot. Note that the lesion is on the contralateral side to the sagging pelvis (on the side of the stance leg). A positive Trendelenburg sign is found in dislocation of the hip, abductor weakness, and shortening of the femoral neck (figure 12.6).
  - ◆ Gowers' sign: Ask the child to get up from squatting position on the floor. With hip and thigh muscle weakness, the child will be unable to stand independently and will use their hands and

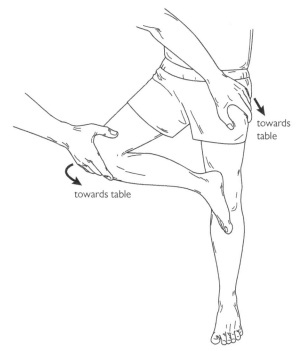

towards
table

towards table

Figure 12.4 FABER test.

arms to 'walk' up the body from a squatting position. In extreme weakness, the child may roll over to the front and 'crawl' up the thighs with their hands to standing position. This is classically seen in proximal muscle weakness (muscular dystrophy, juvenile dermatomyositis).

Knee

With the child lying on the couch:

- Look:
  - from the end of the table for alignment deformity (valgus, lateral malalignment of lower leg, varus, medial malalignment), quadriceps muscle wasting, effusion (absence of normal hollows around the patella), scars, and popliteal fossa swelling
  - from the side for fixed flexion deformity.
- Feel:
  - Assess skin temperature.
  - With the knee slightly flexed, palpate the joint line and the borders of the patella.
  - Palpate the suprapatellar pouch on each side of the quadriceps between the thumb and the fingers for thickening and tenderness of the synovial membrane.
  - Feel the popliteal fossa with the finger tips of both hands.
- Move:
  - Assess full flexion and extension (actively and passively).
  - Assess stability of the knee:
    - Valgus stress to check the medial collateral ligament: slightly flex the knee, place the contralateral hand on the lateral side of the knee, grasp the ankle with the ipsilateral hand and abduct the lower leg. Watch for the degree of motion.

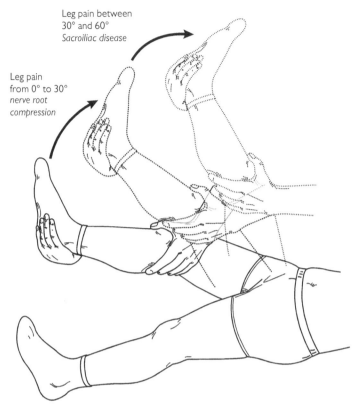

Leg pain between
30° and 60°
Sacroiliac disease

Leg pain
from 0° to 30°
*nerve root
compression*

Figure 12.5 Straight leg raising test.

- Varus stress to check the lateral collateral ligament: slightly flex the knee, place the contralateral hand on the medial side of the knee, grasp the ankle with the ipsilateral hand and adduct the lower leg. Watch for the degree of motion.
- Anterior and posterior draw test: sit at the child's foot, flex the knee to 90°, place the hands on the lower leg with thumbs on the tibia near tibial tuberosity and fingers on the calf muscles, and pull it anteriorly and posteriorly to assess for laxity of the respective cruciate ligaments. Any movement beyond 5 mm suggests ligament laxity.
- McMurray test for meniscal injury: flex the child's hip and knee to 90° with the foot flat on the table. Hold the heel with the right hand and steady the knee with the thumb and index finger of the left hand on either side of the joint. Extend the knee slowly using the right hand and, at the same time, palpate the joint line with the left hand. Repeat this manoeuvre with the tibia in external (rotate the foot and lower leg laterally) and then internal (rotate the foot and lower leg medially) rotation at the various stages of flexion. A positive test is when a 'clunk' is felt with associated pain.
- Joint-specific tests:
  - Patellar tap: extend the knee and squeeze out the suprapatellar pouch by applying pressure with the index finger and the thumb above the knee. While maintaining the pressure, with the tips of the fingers of the free hand, hit the patella downwards with force. If effusion is present, then the patella can be felt striking the femur with a click and bouncing off.
  - Bulge test: useful to identify a small amount of effusion, which may not be identified by patellar tap. Extend the knee and massage the medial aspect of the knee joint upwards with the palm

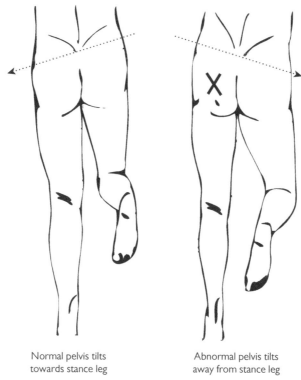

Normal pelvis tilts
towards stance leg

Abnormal pelvis tilts
away from stance leg

Figure 12.6 Trendelenburg's test.

of the hand. Tap the lateral side of the joint at the suprapatellar pouch. Look for a fluid impulse in the medial aspect of the knee.

With the child standing:
- Look:
    - knock-knee (genu valgum)
    - bowleg deformity (genu varum).
- Assessment of function:
    - assess gait (see above).

Foot and ankle

With the child lying on the couch:

- Look:
    - dorsal and plantar surfaces of the foot for deformity, swelling, and nodules
    - alignment deformity such as claw toe or hammertoe
    - nails, nail folds, and between the web spaces
    - the child's shoes.
- Feel:
    - Assess skin temperature.
    - Squeeze the forefoot between thumb and fingers at the level of the metatarsal phalangeal joints.
    - With the thumbs on the sole of foot and the fingers on the dorsum of the foot, palpate the proximal and distal interphalangeal joints and midfoot.

- Palpate anterior surface and joint line of ankle joint, subtalar joint, and origin of plantar fascia into calcaneus.
- Palpate Achilles' tendon for tendonitis and enthesitis (inflamed sites of insertion of tendon). Enthesitis-related arthritis may occur alone or be associated with psoriatic arthritis and HLA B27-related arthritis. Common sites are heel, patella, tibial tuberosity, ischial tuberosity, and sacroiliitis.
- Palpate for peripheral pulses.
- Move:
  - Assess movement actively:
    - Dorsiflexion: 'Lift your foot up'.
    - Plantar flexion: 'Lift your foot up'.
    - 'Curl and extend your toes and then 'cup' the arch of your foot'.
  - Assess movement passively:
    - Dorsiflexion: put one hand on the heel while the ipsilateral forearm supports the foot. Support the tibia with the other hand. Dorsiflex the ankle by lifting the forearm under the foot.
    - Plantar flexion: hold the dorsum of the foot with one hand. Support the tibia with the other hand. Plantar flex the ankle.
    - Inversion and eversion: hold the calcaneus with one hand and the talar neck with the thumb and index finger of the other hand. Apply abducting force (valgus stress) and adducting force (varus stress) with the hand on the calcaneus. Feel the movement of the talus. Holding the talus rather than the tibia isolates subtalar from ankle motion.
    - Rotation at midtarsal joints: hold the calcaneus with one hand and move the forefoot medially and laterally with the other hand.

With the child standing:

- Look:
  - forefoot, midfoot (foot arch), and the hindfoot
  - swelling around the heel and Achilles' tendon
  - ask the child to stand on tiptoes to assess for correction of flatfeet and valgus hind foot
  - ask the child to stand on the outside of foot; stand on inside of foot (neurological and hind foot assessment)
  - assess the gait cycle (heel strike, stance, toe-off).

Spine

- Look:
  - Inspection from behind:
    - scoliosis
    - symmetrical muscle bulk
    - level of iliac crest
    - feet width apart; assess whether the lateral lumbar indentations, dimples of Venus, are at equal height
    - unequal buttock creases.
  - Inspection from the side:
    - normal curvatures: cervical lordosis; thoracic kyphosis; lumbar lordosis.
- Feel:
  - Palpate and percuss spinous processes and intervertebral spaces for tenderness.
  - Palpate paravertebral muscles for spasm or tenderness.

- Move:
  - ◆ Cervical spine:
    - ▪ Extension: 'Look at the roof'.
    - ▪ Flexion: 'Bend your head forward, chin to the chest'.
    - ▪ Rotation: 'Look over each shoulder'.
    - ▪ Lateral flexion at neck: 'Touch each shoulder with your ear'.
  - ◆ Thoracic spine:
    - ▪ Lateral flexion: 'Bend to the right and then left'.
    - ▪ Flexion: 'Bend your back'.
    - ▪ Rotation: 'Twist shoulders to right then left'.
  - ◆ Lumbosacral spine:
    - ▪ Forward flexion at lumbar spine and hip: 'Can you bend to touch your toes?'
    - ▪ Extension: 'Hyperextend at the waist as far as possible'.
    - ▪ Lateral flexion: 'Bend to the right and then left side to side as far as possible at the waist'.
    - ▪ Rotation: 'Look behind by rotating at the waist, while standing steadily (to stabilize the pelvis)'.
    - ▪ Finger excursion: place two fingers on the lumbar vertebrae—the fingers should move apart as the child flexes forwards.
  - ◆ Gait: see above.
  - ◆ Joint-specific test:
    - ▪ Straight leg raising test: see above.
    - ▪ Axial compression test (for cervical radicular pain or paresthesia): forcibly press down vertically on the top of the head with the neck in a neutral position to compress the cervical nerve roots. The test is positive if the pain is exacerbated. Avoid doing this test in children with serious spine disease.
    - ▪ Spurling's test: first extend the neck and compress the head vertically. Next, rotate the head to either side while still extended and apply compression. The test is positive if pain is exacerbated by this position.
    - ▪ Modified Shober's test (to detect and quantify restrictions of lumbar flexion): with the child standing, locate posterior iliac spines (indicated by the dimples of Venus) and mark over the spine at their level. From this line, make a second mark 10 cm superiorly. With the tape in place, ask the child to bend over and attempt to touch their toes. Note down the maximum distance between the two marks and calculate the excursion. Normal excursion is 5–7 cm.
    - ▪ Braggard's test for sciatica: with the knee extended, hold the child's leg and raise it slowly until pain is felt. Lower the leg slightly and dorsiflex the foot briskly. The test is positive if it produces pain in the spine.

Other systems

- Vital signs, especially the temperature chart, blood pressure, dip stick urine.
- Integuments: skin, hair, and nails.
- Eyes for signs of uveitis, cataract, lens dislocation, sclera discoloration.
- System signs and symptoms, for example lymphadenopathy, hepatosplenomegaly, weight loss, night sweats.
- Chest and abdomen for cardiopulmonary or renal involvement.
- Brief neurovascular assessment.

Chapter 13 **Examination of the child with short stature**

Assessment of a child with short stature is one of the commonest endocrinology cases seen in the exam. It is important to remember that short stature is not a disease by itself and is an impairment of linear growth. The term 'short stature' is restricted to height-related issues above 2 years of age, in contrast to 'faltering growth' which focuses on weight related issues in those less than 2 years. Short stature is a height which is less than the third percentile for age on the growth chart derived from local data. Other definitions of impaired linear growth are height significantly below genetic potentials (−2 standard deviations below midparental height), abnormally slow growth velocity, and downwardly crossing percentile channels in a child older than 18 months. To determine the normalcy of stature, one needs a relevant history and serial height measurements over time documented on a growth chart. In the exam, the examiner may provide the context of the case and the child's growth chart. In the United Kingdom, the most widely used charts include the one published by the Child Growth Foundation 1996/1, and the UK–WHO growth charts published by the Royal College of Paediatrics and Child Health using the World Health Organization standards (figure 13.1). Be familiar with the use of the different charts and remember to use growth charts appropriate for sex and underlying disease (Down's syndrome, Turner's syndrome). The causes of short stature are given in table 13.1 and features of common conditions causing short stature in table 13.2. Possible conditions seen in a child with short stature commonly encountered in the MRCPCH Clinical Exam are listed in table 13.3.

You may be asked to assess the child's growth or assess the child with short stature. Such an assessment is appropriate only after taking into account the history and physical examination findings. However, in the clinical exam, you will not be allowed to take a history and have to evaluate the child based on the clues available at the bedside and examination findings.

General approach

These steps are repeated in every system to reiterate their importance and to help you recollect the initial approach of any clinical exam. Also refer to chapter 4.

- *On entering the examination room, demonstrate strict adherence to infection control measures by washing your hands or by using alcohol rub.*
- Introduce yourself *both* to the parents and the child.
- Talk slowly and clearly with a smile on your face.
- Establish rapport with the child and parents.
- Find out the *age* of the child, if not told already.
- Confirm the relationship of the adult who is present with the child.
- Expose adequately while ensuring the child's privacy. The child should be sufficiently undressed, but draped with underwear and gown to preserve modesty. Be careful with teenagers, who might resent being in minimal clothing. For examination of the limbs, expose both the upper and lower limbs.
- Positioning: child should be awake and alert and the room should be warm and adequately lit. For assessment, the older child should be standing on the floor. Initial examination of a toddler can be done on the parent's lap rather than on a couch. Later, after establishing rapport, the child should stand alone for measurements and manoeuvres.

Examination of the child with short stature comprises of four stages: head to toe visual survey, measurements, manoeuvres and systemic examination.

Visual survey—head to toe examination

Take a few seconds to watch the child actively, from head to toe, at the start and make observations on the well-being of the child and their interactions. Look for both obvious and subtle dysmorphic features, which might fit into a recognizable syndrome. Do not ignore items in their immediate vicinity.

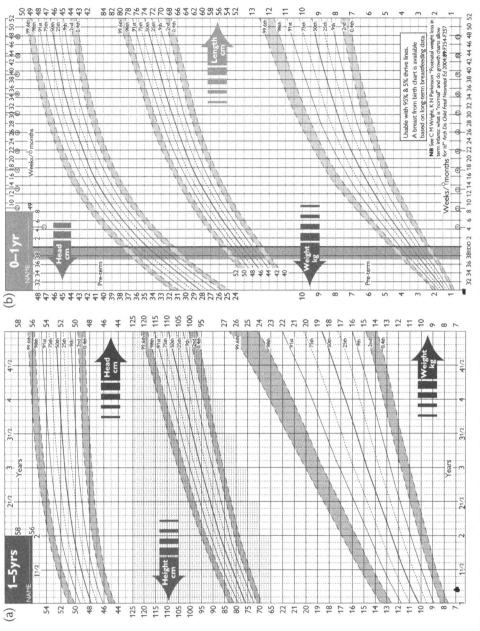

Figure 13.1 Growth charts for (a) boys between 1 and 5 years and (b) girls between 0 and 1 year. Reproduced with permission from the Child Growth Foundation.

Table 13.1 Causes of short stature

Growth hormone deficient

Idiopathic

Organic causes
  Congenital, e.g. septo-optic dysplasia
  Empty sella syndrome
  Pituitary/hypothalamic tumour, e.g. craniopharyngiomas
  Cranial irradiation
  Other acquired, e.g. trauma, meningitis, or encephalitis

Non-growth hormone deficient

Familial short stature

Constitutional delay

Intrauterine growth restriction

Syndromes
  Down's syndrome
  Turner's syndrome
  Noonan's syndrome
  Prader–Willi syndrome
  IUGR-related syndromes (Russell–Silver syndrome)

Diseases of other systems
  Cardiac
  Renal
  Respiratory (cystic fibrosis)
  Malnutrition
  Malabsorption (inflammatory bowel disease, coeliac disease)

Skeletal dysplasia
  Short limb dwarfism, e.g. achondroplasia, hypochondroplasia
  Osteogenesis imperfecta
  Mucopolysaccharidosis
  Mucolipidosis

Endocrine disorders
  Hypothyroidism
  Cushing's syndrome
  Precocious puberty

Social deprivation

- Comment on the following:
  - state of wakefulness: awake/aware/alert/active
  - general well-being: well, ill
  - attention, behaviour, interest in the surroundings, play, relation with parents
  - looks: normal or syndromic
  - growth: see next section, personal health record of the child (the Red Book), if available
  - development: Tanner staging for pubertal development in teenagers should be recorded.
  - Body habitus:
    - Overweight, plethoric, striae; kyphosis suggests Cushing's syndrome.
    - Disproportionate body proportions imply skeletal dysplasias.

Table 13.2 Features of common conditions causing short stature

Familial short stature	Height below the 3rd centile but appropriate for parental heights
	Steady growth below, but parallel to, the normal growth curves
	At least one parent is short
	Puberty occurs at the normal age compared to peers
	Bone age is consistent with chronological age
Constitutional growth delay	Short stature
	Reduced growth velocity during the first 3 years, with normal growth velocity thereafter
	Delayed sexual maturation
	Delayed bone age
	More common in boys
	Family history of delay
	Final adult height usually within the normal range
	May benefit from treatment with gonadal steroids
Intrauterine growth restriction	Height below the 3rd centile and small for parental heights
	Steady growth below but parallel to the normal growth curves
	Some children might have catch up growth
	Parents usually have normal height
	Puberty occurs at the normal age compared to peers
	Bone age is consistent with chronological age
Growth hormone deficiency	Short stature with proportionate body
	Facial phenotype resembling a younger child
	Increased subcutaneous fat
	Frontal bossing
	Midfacial hypoplasia
	Microphallus in boys
	Subnormal growth velocity
	Delayed bone age
Hypothyroidism	Short stature
	Delayed bone age
	Delayed sexual maturation
	Decreased growth velocity
	Dry skin, constipation, cold intolerance
Cushing's syndrome	Slow growth velocity
	Delayed bone age relative to the chronological age
	Excessive weight gain and truncal obesity
	Elevated blood pressure
Psychosocial deprivation	Poor growth
	Withdrawn child who avoids eye contact
	Bizarre behaviour, poor speech and language development
	Increased growth velocity in a more secure environment

- Decreased weight for height is seen in malnutrition from any cause.
- Loss of fat and muscle mass with shrunken, wasted appearance is seen in protein energy malnutrition.
- Loss of secondary sexual characteristics in a female suggests an eating disorder, such as anorexia nervosa.

Table 13.3 Conditions involving short stature that may be seen in the MRCPCH Clinical Exam

Endocrine	Hypothyroidism
	Pseudohypoparathyroidism
	Cushing's syndrome
Syndromes	Down's syndrome
	Turner's syndrome
	Noonan's syndrome
	Williams' syndrome
	Russell–Silver syndrome
Chronic diseases	Chronic renal failure
	Post-renal transplant
	Cyanotic congenital heart disease
	Chronic juvenile arthritis
	Crohn's disease
	Ulcerative colitis
	Cystic fibrosis
Skeletal dysplasia	Achondroplasia
	Spondyloepiphyseal dysplasia
Iatrogenic	Chronic steroid use—Cushing's syndrome
	Spinal irradiation
	Post-intracranial surgery
Miscellaneous	Familial short stature
	Constitutional growth failure

- Head:
  - size: microcephaly (TORCH, Seckel's syndrome, Williams' syndrome), macrocephaly (achondroplasia, hydrocephalus)
  - shape: brachycephaly (Down's syndrome), occipital protuberance (Dandy–Walker malformation), frontal bossing with macrocephaly (achondroplasia), dolichocephaly (preterm).
- Face:
  - shape: small triangular face and micrognathia (Russell–Silver syndrome), triangular face (Noonan's syndrome), micrognathia (Seckel's syndrome), moon face (Cushing's syndrome).
  - dysmorphic features: midfacial abnormalities (clefts, bifid uvula, maxillary incisor, hypoplasia, seen in pituitary abnormality and growth hormone deficiency), coarse features (glycogen storage disorder and, rarely, hypothyroidism), upturned nose, long philtrum with micrognathia (Williams' syndrome), smooth philtrum, thin vermilion, small palpebral fissures (fetal alcohol syndrome), flattened nose, small mouth, protruding tongue, small ears, upward slanting eyes, epicanthal fold (Down's syndrome).
- Eye:
  - visual field examination and fundoscopy: papilloedema, optic atrophy (underlying CNS disease causing growth hormone deficiency).
- Neck:
  - webbed neck: Turner's syndrome, Noonan's syndrome
  - goitre: hypothyroidism
  - bitemporal hemianopia: pituitary or hypothalamic lesions (craniopharyngioma).

- Skin:
  - acne, facial hair: Cushing's syndrome
  - scars.
- Hands:
  - clubbing: Crohn's disease, ulcerative colitis, cystic fibrosis, congenital cyanotic heart disease.

Measurements

Measurements play an important part in the assessment of a child with short stature.

- Child:
  - **Height**: recumbent length is plotted for children up to 24 months of age using a Harpenden infantometer. The infantometer consists of a flat surface with a fixed headboard and movable base plate. The child is placed on the back and head is held in position at the fixed end by one observer. The movable foot piece is brought up to the feet by a second assistant, who should ensure the body, legs, and feet are in a straight line, and the length is measured. In children older than 2 years, standing height is measured using the stadiometer. Ask the child to stand against the wall facing forward with the arms by the side of the body and the feet side by side (figure 13.2). Position the head so that the plane of the eyes is parallel to the ground (Frankfurt plane) and heel, buttock, and the upper back are touching the wall. Accurately measure the height and plot it on an appropriate centile chart.
  - **Lower segment**: next, with the child in the same position, measure the distance from the top of the symphysis pubis to the floor, which will give the lower segment.
  - **Upper segment/lower segment ratio (US/LS ratio)**: calculate the upper segment by subtracting the lower segment from the height and compute the US/LS ratio. This indicates whether the short stature is proportionate (i.e. involves both the trunk and the lower limbs, e.g. short stature due to chronic diseases) or disproportionate (i.e. involves one more than the other, e.g. primary bone disorders). The US/LS ratio decreases progressively from 1.7 at birth until 8 years when it reaches 1. The formula for normal age-appropriate ratio is 1: 1+ (1/age in years).
  - **Arm span**: position the child against a wall, with the feet together, the arms stretched sideways, and the palms facing forwards. Measure the distance between the tips of the middle fingers. Arm span is approximately equal to the height above 8 years of age. Arm span is an indicator of extremity growth and can be used as a surrogate for height measurement in children who have scoliosis or contractures.
  - **Weight and weight for height ratio**: measure the weight using a digital scale. Place the scale on a firm floor rather than carpet. Remove the child's shoes and heavy clothing and ask them to stand with both feet close together in the centre of the scale. Record the weight and determine the weight for height ratio. This ratio is relatively preserved in endocrine disorders (growth hormone deficiency, hypothyroidism and Cushing's disease) in contrast to systemic disorders, which are associated with poor weight gain and linear growth.
- Parent:
  - **Midparental height**: obtain the parents' heights (wherever possible) and plot on the child's chart. Measured parental heights should *always* be obtained as reported heights are notoriously inaccurate. Calculate the midparental percentile (MPC) for boys by adding 7 cm to the mean of the father's and mother's height in cm. For girls, subtract 7 cm from the mean of the heights. The child's target centile range (TCR) is ± 10 cm and ± 8.5 cm of the midparental height for boys and girls, respectively. The midparental height predicts the target height based on the genetic potential and helps to determine if the child's height is appropriate considering the height of the parents.

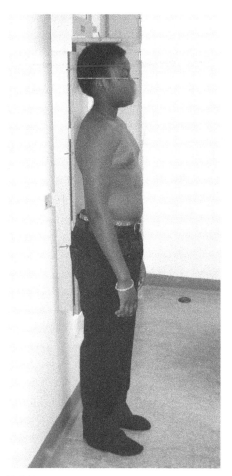

Figure 13.2 Measurement of height.

Frankfurt plan: position of reference in which the upper border of the external auditory meatus is on a horizontal plane with the lower border of the eye.

Manoeuvres

To identify the region that predominately contributes to the short stature and the cause, perform the following sets of manoeuvres. Ask the child to stand upright and observe from the front (figure 13.3).

- Step 1: look at the palms of the hands for clinodactyly (Russell–Silver syndrome, Down's syndrome), single palmar crease (Down's syndrome), swollen wrists (juvenile chronic arthritis), splayed wrists (rickets), polydactyly (Bardet–Biedl syndrome), and bowlegs (rickets).
- Step 2: ask the child to make a fist and turn their hand over to look for shortened fourth metacarpal (pseudohypoparathyroidism, Turner's syndrome, and McCune–Albright syndrome).
- Step 3 screening for unilateral limb shortening (asymmetry): ask the child to stand erect and put their hands and the palms together in the midline without flexion at the elbows, hips or knees (Russell–Silver syndrome).

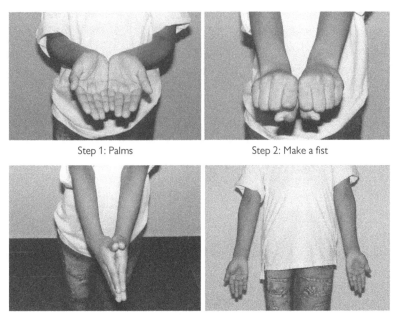

Step 1: Palms   Step 2: Make a fist

Step 3: Hands and palms in midline   Step 4: Carrying angle

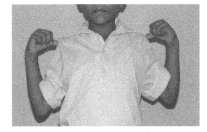

Step 5: Touch shoulders with tip of the thumb

Figure 13.3 Manoeuvres for examination of short stature. See also colour plate section.

- Step 4, carrying angle (angle made by the axes of the arm and the forearm, with the elbow in full extension): ask the child to keep their arms at the sides, extended at the elbow and the palms face forward, and look at the carrying angle. Normal carrying angle is up to 15° (increased in Turner's syndrome).
- Step 5: ask the child to bend their elbow and touch their shoulders with the tip of the thumb on both sides, which normal children should be able to do. In rhizomelic dwarfism (short arms), the thumbs will go beyond the shoulder. In mesomelic (short forearm) and acromelic (short hands) dwarfism, the thumbs will fall short of the shoulder.

Systemic examination

Next, a screening examination of the various regions should be done. Finally, complete examination of the system identified in the screening is performed to identify the cause of short stature.

- Respiratory:
  - pectus excavatum or carinatum: Noonan's syndrome

- shield chest: Turner's syndrome
- hyperinflation: chronic asthma
- crackles: cystic fibrosis.
- Endocrine:
  - slow pulse rate, slow relaxation of the Achilles tendon reflex: hypothyroidism.
- Cardiovascular:
  - bradycardia with hypotension is seen in eating disorders
  - hypertension: kidney disease, Cushing's syndrome
  - cyanosis and clubbing suggests congenital cyanotic heart disease
  - cardiac murmurs are heard in children with congenital heart disease
  - heart failure: congenital acyanotic heart disease.
- Abdominal:
  - abdominal distension: coeliac disease
  - scars: Crohn's disease, ulcerative colitis, and previous abdominal malignancy
  - hepatosplenomegaly is seen in glycogen storage disorder type 1.
- Genitalia:
  - *Ask the child for permission before proceeding to examine the genitalia.* The examiner will usually stop you if there is nothing specific to find in the examination or he or she may ask you what you are going to look for.
  - Look for abnormalities of the genitalia, such as undescended testes and hypospadias in boys and clitoromegaly and fused labia in girls. Penile length and testicular size should be measured.
  - Hypospadias: Russell–Silver syndrome.
  - Microphallus: defect in hypothalamic–pituitary–gonadal axis or in peripheral androgen action. Micropenis may also be caused by isolated growth hormone deficiency.
- Neurological:
  - hypotonia: Prader–Willi syndrome, myopathy.

Chapter 14 **Examination of the skin and skin appendages**

Examination of the skin can provide information about cutaneous or systemic diseases. As always, examination of the skin is best performed in correlation with the available medical history. Even if the examination is conducted in a different order, you should have a systematic method of presenting the findings. Examination comprises inspection and palpation of skin and skin appendages (hair, nails, teeth, and mucous membranes) and is performed in one of two scenarios.

1. The skin may be sequentially examined alongside the examination of other systems (e.g. neurocutaneous syndromes, which are disorders with neurological features, characteristics lesions on the skin, and tumours in different parts of the body) (table 14.1).
2. A dedicated examination of the skin may need to be carried out when it is the suspected primary involved organ and includes evaluation of the hair, nails, teeth, and mucous membranes of the mouth and genitalia.

Key competence skills required in examination of the skin are given in table 14.2. Some of the clinical features of common paediatric dermatoses are given in table 14.3.

General approach

These steps are repeated in every system to reiterate their importance and to help you recollect the initial approach of any clinical exam. Also refer to chapter 4.

- *On entering the examination room, demonstrate strict adherence to infection control measures by washing your hands or by using alcohol rub.*
- Introduce yourself *both* to the parents and the child.
- Talk slowly and clearly with a smile on your face.
- Establish rapport with the child and parents.
- Expose adequately while ensuring their privacy.
- Positioning: the patient must be undressed adequately to carry out a complete examination. Inadequate skin exposure with the cloth pushed to one side or lifted momentarily often casts shadows on the skin and is not conducive for proper examination. Infants and very young children should be undressed completely. The younger child is examined preferably on the parent's lap. Older children can lie down except for the examination of back, which can be examined in the sitting position.
- Lighting: examination of the skin should be performed in an environment with good illumination. The child should be examined in an environment with bright overhead and side lighting. The best source of lighting is natural daylight. Inadequate lighting is the most common cause of an incomplete skin examination. Mobile lighting is required for close inspection of lesions. A torch with a well lit cone is essential for examination of the mouth and transillumination. A hand lens is often useful for detailed examination and *a ruler is essential* for recording the size of lesions. If natural light through a window is used, it is critical to protect the patient's privacy inside the examination room.

Visual survey—head to toe examination

- Look for every possible clue available, which may help you to make the correct diagnosis.
- Look and try to estimate the approximate age of the child.
- Always think whether the findings constitute a recognizable clinical syndrome.
- Every exam candidate is expected to be familiar with dermatological descriptive terms but it is best to describe your findings in plain language.

Table 14.1 Neurocutaneous syndromes

Syndrome	Neurological features	Cutaneous features	Other features
Ataxia telangiectasia	Progressive neurological impairment, cerebellar ataxia, choreoathetosis	Ocular and cutaneous telangiectasia	Autosomal recessive disorder, variable immunodeficiency with susceptibility to sinopulmonary infections, and predisposition to malignancy
Hypomelanosis of Ito	Seizures, learning difficulties, developmental delay, deafness, visual problems	Whirled hypochromic patches along Blaschko lines	Hemihypertrophy, arm and leg length discrepancy, and scoliosis
Incontinentia pigmenti	Seizures, developmental delay, learning difficulties, ataxia, spastic paralysis, microcephaly	Neonatal vesicular rash with eosinophilia, hyperpigmentation on the trunk, fading in adolescence Linear, atrophic, hairless lesions Whorled pattern of lesions	Seen in girls (lethal in boys) Three stages of skin lesions: vesiculobullous, verrucous, pigmentary Ophthalmological (loss of visual acuity, strabismus, optic nerve atrophy, microphthalmia, keratitis, cataracts, iris hypoplasia, nystagmus) and dental manifestations
Linear nevus syndrome	Moderate to severe learning difficulties, developmental delay, hemiparesis, seizures	Linear, verrucous or nodular facial nevus with hyperplastic sebaceous glands, present on the forehead down into the nasal area near the midline	Ocular (esotropia, coloboma of the eyelid, iris or choroid, cloudy cornea, homonymous hemianopia) Renal manifestations (renal hamartomata, nephroblastoma, Wilms' tumour)
Neurofibromatosis type 1	High prevalence of seizures, learning disabilities, attention deficit disorder, and speech problems	Café au lait macules: brown coloured patches may be present at birth and increase in size and number with age Axillary or inguinal freckling develops by 3 years Cutaneous and plexiform neurofibromas develop during puberty	Bone deformities also may develop Lisch nodules (found on the iris of the eye)
Sturge–Weber syndrome	Epilepsy, learning difficulties, hemiplegia, ipsilateral leptomeningeal angioma	Multiple angiomas involving the face, eye, and brain Port-wine stain (non-elevated capillary angioma) present in the ophthalmic branch of the trigeminal nerve distribution Usually unilateral	Sporadic condition May manifest with glaucoma
Tuberous sclerosis	Seizures, behavioural problems, learning difficulties	Periungual fibromas, cutaneous angiofibromas (adenoma sebaceum) from 5 years, mainly affecting the centre of the face, Shagreen patches (brown leathery thickenings of the skin) and ash leaf macules (depigmented)	Hamartomas in brain, kidneys, heart, eyes, lungs, and skin Variable expression and penetrance
Von Hippel–Lindau disease	Tumours of the central nervous system	Café au lait spots, angiomatosis	Haemangioblastomas, phaeochromocytoma, renal cell carcinoma, and pancreatic cysts

Table 14.2 Key competence skills required in examination of the skin

Competence skill	Standard
Knowledge of dermatological descriptive terms	Ability to describe skin rashes and lesions in simple language
	Ability to apply appropriate descriptive dermatological terms
Understanding that hair, teeth, and nail are appendages of the skin	Look for clinical evidence of associated hair, teeth, and nail involvement
Clear understanding that skin conditions may be part of a neurocutaneous syndrome	Ability to recognize skin lesions with associated underlying neurological conditions such as café au lait spots with neurofibromatosis type1, port-wine stain in Sturge–Weber syndrome, ash leaf macules in tuberous sclerosis
Understanding that skin conditions may have underlying systemic causes	Ability to identify and diagnose underlying systemic involvement
Recognition of common skin rashes	Ability to recognize quickly common rashes in children such as atopic eczema, seborrhoeic dermatitis, infection, infestation, and common rashes
Recognition of malignant conditions of the skin and conditions which later develop into malignancy in children	Ability to identify and accurately describe skin malignancy such as malignant melanoma or premalignant conditions such as dysplastic naevus syndromes and giant melanocytic naevus

- Comment on the following:
  - state of wakefulness
  - general well being
  - interest in the surroundings
  - growth of the child
  - environment (equipment)
  - head
  - face
  - teeth
  - hands.

  Proceed to specific inspection of the skin.

Examination of the skin

Inspection

Start with a general observation of the skin. This is followed by inspection of the individual lesions, which are best described by the ABCDE rule (Asymmetry of the lesion, Border irregularity, Colour of the lesion including uniformity of the pigmentation, Diameter and distribution, Edge). Other points to include are location, number (isolated and well localized or coalescent and diffuse), shape (oval, circular, annular), appearance (similar or monomorphic, different or pleomorphic), level with the surrounding skin (flat, raised above the surface, depressed), consistency (solid, fluid filled), and type of lesion (primary or secondary) (tables 14.4 and 14.5).

Primary lesions are the initial lesions in the skin caused directly by the disease process, while secondary lesions evolve from primary lesions having been modified by external forces such as scratching, picking, infection, or healing (table 14.6, figures 14.1, 14.2, and 14.3).

Table 14.3 Diagnosis of common paediatric dermatosis

Condition	Morphological appearance of lesions	Distribution of lesions	Arrangement of lesions	Number of lesions
Acne	Areas of skin with non-inflammatory follicular papules or comedones Inflammatory papules, pustules, and nodules in more severe forms	Face and other parts of the skin that contain the highest concentration of sebaceous glands	None specific	Depends on severity
Addison's disease	Hyperpigmentation	Most visible on scars, skin folds, pressure points such as the elbows, knees, knuckles and toes, lips, buccal mucosa, and photo-exposed areas		
Allergic contact dermatitis	Pruritic papules and vesicles on an erythematous base	Exposed areas with localized distribution	Linear lesions in areas of contact	Depends on exposure and severity
Atopic dermatitis	Acute: intensely pruritic vesicles and blisters with intense erythema Subacute: pruritic eczematous lesions with erythema, scaling, and fissuring of the skin Chronic: thickened skin, accentuated skin lines, excoriations and fissuring accompanying a moderate to intense itch	Face, flexures of arms and legs (antecubital fossae and popliteal fossae), wrists, nipples and eyelids in infants, extensor surface in younger children, flexor aspect in older children	Bilaterally symmetrical	Varies
Candidiasis	Pruritic, well-demarcated, erythematous patches of varying size and shape Satellite papules and pustules adjacent to primary patches	Intertriginous areas such as axilla, neck, groin, and gluteal folds, web spaces of fingers and toes, glans penis and beneath the breasts		
Chronic bullous disease of childhood	Pruritic tense blisters over red base	Genitalia, periorificial, perioral lesions	New blisters developing around the healed ones String of pearl appearance	
Dermatitis herpetiformis	Intensely itchy, polymorphic papulovesicular eruptions	Extensor surfaces (buttocks, back of neck, scalp, elbows, knees, back)	Symmetrical distribution	
Dermatomyositis	Heliotrope rash (violaceous to dusky erythematous rash with or without oedema), Gottron papules (slightly elevated, violaceous papules and plaques over bony prominences), periungual telangiectasia	Periorbital, heliotrope rash, central face and scalp	Symmetrical distribution of heliotrope rash	

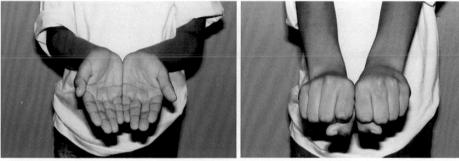

Step 1: Palms

Step 2: Make a fist

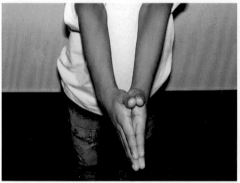

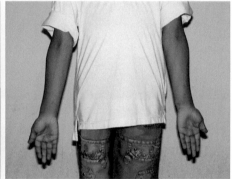

Step 3: Hands and palms in midline

Step 4: Carrying angle

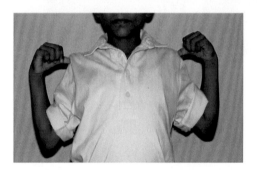

Step 5: Touch shoulders with tip of the thumb

Figure 13.3 Manoeuvres for examination of short stature.

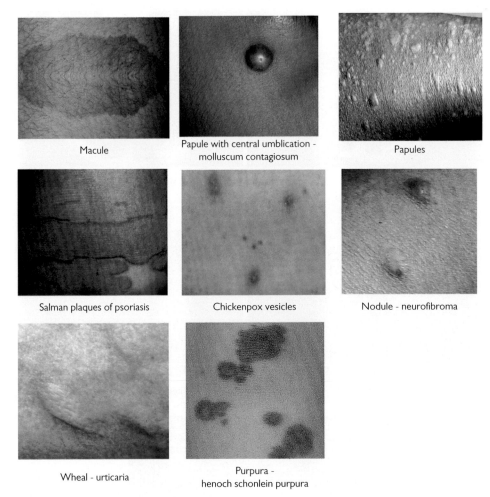

Macule

Papule with central umblication - molluscum contagiosum

Papules

Salman plaques of psoriasis

Chickenpox vesicles

Nodule - neurofibroma

Wheal - urticaria

Purpura - henoch schonlein purpura

Figure 14.1 Primary lesions of the skin.

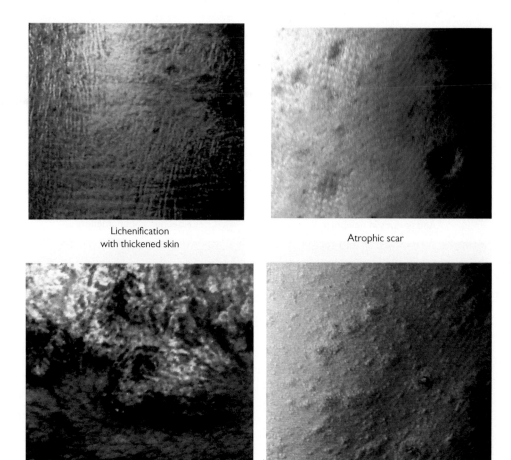

Lichenification
with thickened skin

Atrophic scar

Silvery scales of psoriasis

Peripheral scaling - pityriasis rosea

Figure 14.2 Secondary lesions of the skin.

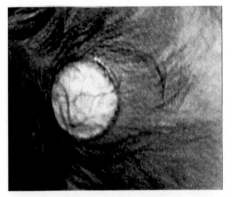

Aplasia cutis in newborn

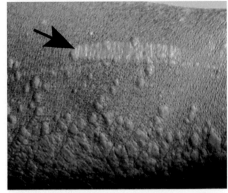

Koebner's phenomenon

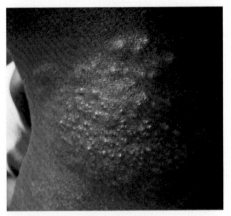

Clustered vesicles -
herpes zoster

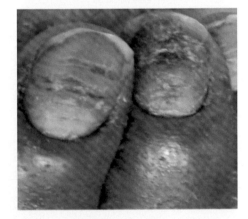

Thickening and ridges -
nail psoriasis

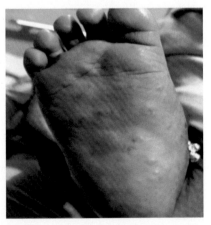

Papular acrodermatitis

Figure 14.3 More examples of cutaneous lesions.

Table 14.3 *Continued*

Condition	Morphological appearance of lesions	Distribution of lesions	Arrangement of lesions	Number of lesions
Erythema nodosum	Red shiny lumps 1–3 cm in diameter Initially purple and painful	Distributed over the front of the shins		
Erythema multiforme	Polymorphic eruption: erythematous, expanding macules or papules evolve into target lesions, with bright red borders and central petechiae, vesicles or purpura	Palms and dorsum of the hands, soles, extensor surface of extremities, face Mucous membrane involved in severe cases	Symmetrical distribution	
Epidermolysis bullosa	Blisters may present with old scars Nails are dysplastic	Over both knees		
Factitious illness	Similar looking lesions	Areas of skin accessible to manipulation (e.g. the posterior shoulders but not the middle of the back)	Predominantly on the left side in right handed patient and vice versa in left handed patients	Varies
Henoch–Schönlein purpura	Palpable purpura, oedema of hands, feet and scalp	Typically on the legs and buttocks, but may also be seen on the arms, face, and trunk		
Herpes zoster	Vesicular rash over erythematous base, markedly tender	Dermatomal	Clustered	
Kawasaki's disease	Maculopapular erythematous lesions, urticariform type rash, erythema multiforme Peeling of the skin in the genital area, hands, and feet in later phases	Hands and feet	Symmetrical distribution	
Phototoxic drug eruptions	Various types	Sun-exposed areas of the body		
Psoriasis	Red, scaly patches	Scalp, extensor aspect of arms and legs, umbilicus, gluteal cleft and fingernails Lesions can involve the entire body surface Pitting nails	Often symmetrical Koebner phenomenon	Number of lesions is an indication of the severity
Seborrhoeic dermatitis	Greasy scaling over red, inflamed skin presenting as patchy scaling to widespread, thick, adherent crusts	Sebum rich areas of the scalp, face, and trunk		
Scabies (unlikely in exam)	Burrows	Interdigital areas, genitalia		

Table 14.4 Regional distribution of paediatric skin diseases

Face	Infantile eczema, Sturge–Weber syndrome, dermatomyositis, scabies in infants
Mouth	Candidiasis, herpes simplex, Peutz–Jeghers syndrome, xanthelasma (hyperlipidaemia)
Trunk	Most viral rashes, neurofibromatosis, herpes zoster (dermatome distribution), Addison's (areolar and scar pigmentation), erythema multiforme, pityriasis rosea
Elbow	Atopic eczema (extensor in younger and flexor in older child), xanthomata (extensor), phrynoderma
Hands	Kawasaki's disease (red and swollen or peeling skin), Addison's (skin crease pigmentation), scabies (interdigital areas), dermatomyositis, erythema multiforme (polymorphic eruption, macules, vesicles, bullae), verruca vulgaris
Nails	Psoriasis (pitting nails), iron deficiency (koilonychia), fungal dystrophy
Legs	Necrobiosis lipoidica diabeticorum, pretibial myxoedema, erythema nodosum, Henoch–Schönlein purpura (extensor aspects ankles and buttocks), xanthomata in Achilles, tendon
Feet	Verrucae, Kawasaki (swelling or peeling), pustular psoriasis, eczema, phrynoderma
Buttocks and elbows	Dermatitis herpetiformis
Genitalia and perioral lesions	Chronic bullous disease of childhood, acrodermatitis enteropathica
Dermatomal	Herpes zoster

- **Skin colour**: while describing the colour, one should decide if it correlates with the race. Generalized hypopigmentation is seen in albinism and phenylketonuria. Yellow discoloration of the skin is seen in jaundice (involving the mucosa and the sclera) or hypercarotinaemia (sparing mucosa and the sclera). Ashen grey or pale skin is seen in shock. Generalized hyperpigmentation is seen in Addison's disease and haemosiderosis.
- **Localized pigmentation**: may present as hyperpigmentation (skin naevi) or hypopigmentation (postinflammatory lesions, pityriasis alba, tinea versicolor, ash leaf macules in tuberous sclerosis, hypomelanosis of Ito or vitiligo).
- Inspect all areas including nails, mucous membranes, scalp, axilla, buttocks, and perineum as follows (figures 14.4 and 14.5).
   - Step 1: start with the face, giving special attention to the nose, lips, mouth (gums, tongue, and buccal mucosa), eyelids, and dorsal and ventral surface of the ears.
   - Step 2: proceed to inspect thoroughly the scalp, hair shaft, and the hair root.
   - Step 3: examine the palm and the dorsum of the hands carefully, paying particular attention to the skin between fingers and the area beneath the fingernails.
   - Step 4: continue up the wrists and examine both front and back of the forearm. Next move to the elbows and look at the arms including the axilla.
   - Step 5: focus on the neck, the chest, and the abdomen. With adolescent girls, carefully examine the under surface of the breasts (or at least say that you would examine the skin beneath the breasts).
   - Step 6: inspect the dorsal surface of the neck, shoulders, and the back including the buttocks.
   - Step 7: move onto the lower limb and look at the anterior and posterior surface of both thighs and legs, the dorsal and ventral aspects of the foot, between the toes, and under toenails.
   - Step 8: last but not the least is the examination of the genital region. In general, this is avoided in the exam, but it is important to mention to the examiner.

Table 14.5 Descriptive terms in dermatology

Term	Definition
Annular ring	Ring-shaped lesion with dark edge and central clearing
Arcuate	Incomplete circle
Clustered	Multiple lesions grouped within an area
Digitate	Finger shaped
Discoid/nummular	Filled circle, coin like
Discrete	Lesions separated by normal skin
Disseminated	Widespread, discrete lesions
Eczematoid	Inflamed lesions with a tendency towards oozing or crusting
Erythema	Redness due to capillary dilation that blanches on pressure
Follicular	Lesions involving the hair follicle
Friable	Surface bleeds easily after minor trauma
Generalized	Covering most of body, without intervening normal skin
Guttate	Drop like
Indurated	Abnormal hardening skin cannot be pinched over the lesions
Koebner phenomenon	Reproduction of skin lesions at sites of trauma
Linear	Arranged in a line
Livedo	Lesions in a hatched pattern
Multiform	Presence of lesions of variety of shapes
Papillomatous/warty	Finger-like or round projections from surface of the lesion
Pedunculated	Lesion with a stalk having a narrower diameter at the base
Photodistribution	Lesions occurring over sun exposed skin
Reticulate	Fine, net-like pattern
Scarlatiniform	Innumerable small red papules that are widely and diffusely distributed
Serpiginous	Snake shaped
Stellate	Star shaped
Target	Lesions presenting as concentric rings
Umbilicated	Elevated lesion with central depression
Zosteriform	Lesions follow a dermatome

Palpation

Ensure that your hands are warm before palpation. Gloves are not necessary when examining intact skin. Non-latex gloves should be worn when you examine broken skin and mucous membranes.

- Step 1 **general palpation of the skin**, in particular the uninvolved areas. Points to note while palpating are coarseness of the skin and skin temperature.
- Step 2 **palpation of the individual lesions**:
    - tenderness
    - surface
    - depth of involvement of the skin or subcutis

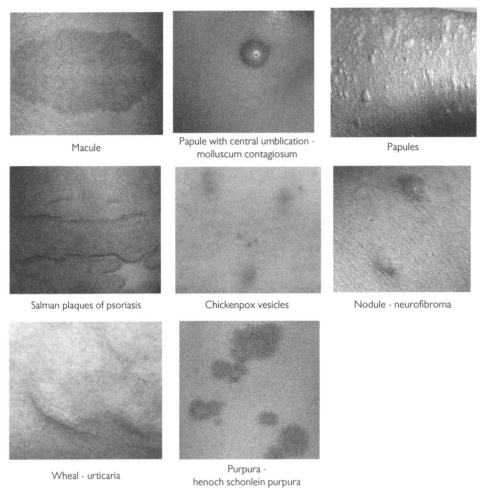

Macule

Papule with central umblication -
molluscum contagiosum

Papules

Salman plaques of psoriasis

Chickenpox vesicles

Nodule - neurofibroma

Wheal - urticaria

Purpura -
henoch schonlein purpura

Figure 14.1 Primary lesions of the skin. See also colour plate section.

- ◆ texture of the lesion (firm or soft)
- ◆ thickness of lesions above the surface of skin
- ◆ mobility of the lesion from underlying structures
- ◆ presence, texture, and quantity of scales. Do the scales flake off easily?
- ◆ in crusted lesions, determine what is beneath the crust.
- Step 3 **squeeze the skin**: a dimple will appear with dermatofibromas.
- Step 4 **surrounding skin**: stroke the skin linearly with pressure (to elicit dermographism) and apply tangential pressure on perilesional skin (to elicit Nikolsky's sign, which is present when slight rubbing of the skin results in exfoliation of the skin's outermost layer). Nikolsky's sign is seen in pemphigus, toxic epidermal necrolysis, and staphylococcal scalded skin syndrome.
- Step 5 **diascopy**: apply vertical pressure with a transparent glass slide and squeeze the blood out of the skin to enhance the visibility of the lesions. Diascopy is useful in distinguishing intravascular (erythema) and extravasated blood (purpura). This is a useful sign to distinguish meningococcal purpura from viral rashes, which fade on pressure.

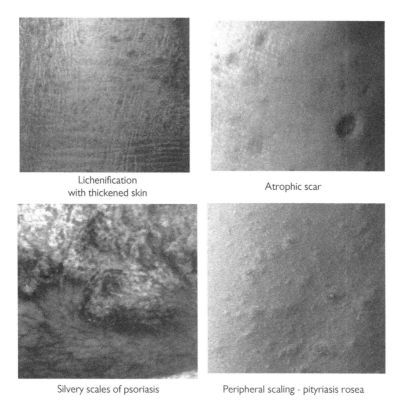

Lichenification with thickened skin

Atrophic scar

Silvery scales of psoriasis

Peripheral scaling - pityriasis rosea

Figure 14.2 Secondary lesions of the skin. See also colour plate section.

Examination of the hair

Examination of the hair in the scalp, axilla, and body is part of skin examination. As usual, this starts with **inspection** of the hair. Points to note during inspection are:

- quantity and density of hair: excess/sparse/absence of hair
- site of hair loss or excess: generalized or localized
- length of hair
- colour of hair
- texture (straight, wavy, or curly)
- skin in areas of hair loss: look for scarring (absence of follicles), erythema, scaling, excoriation
- presence of nits (egg cases of lice).
  After inspection, proceed to **palpation** of the hair.
- Hair pull test: identifies excess hair shedding. Grasp a tuft of hair and pull the tuft firmly, but gently. Normally, up to two hairs can be extracted. Examine the pulled out hair under a magnifying glass. Presence of a rounded bulb at the proximal end suggests that the hair is telogen hair, while anagen hair will have a tapered end.

Examination of the nails

Even though the nails can provide valuable information about systemic and cutaneous diseases, examination of the nails is often ignored. Nail abnormalities can present with problems of the colour,

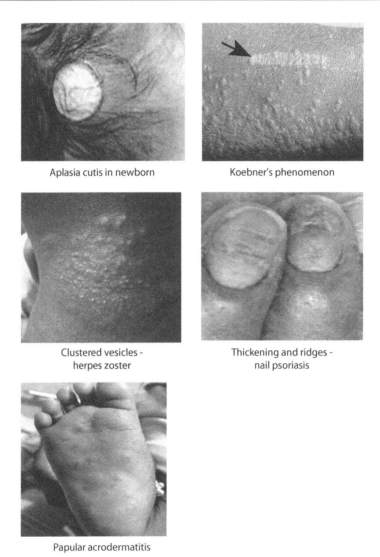

Aplasia cutis in newborn

Koebner's phenomenon

Clustered vesicles -
herpes zoster

Thickening and ridges -
nail psoriasis

Papular acrodermatitis

Figure 14.3 More examples of cutaneous lesions. See also colour plate section.

shape, texture, or thickness of the nail plate or cuticle. Nails should be systematically examined as follows.

- Step 1 **nail plate**:
  - ◆ Surface:
    - ■ Look for the **presence of a nail plate** in all the fingers. Loss of nail plate can be congenital or secondary to trauma or severe systemic illness. In nail–patella syndrome, the nail plate is typically absent on the thumb and, even when present, it never reaches the free edge of the finger.
    - ■ **Pitting** of nails (presence of small depressions on the nail surface) can be seen in eczema, psoriasis, ectodermal dysplasia, and alopecia areata (Figure 14.3).

Table 14.6 Primary and secondary lesions of the skin

Name	Description	Example
Primary lesion		
Macule	Flat, non-palpable area of altered colour of the skin	Freckles, nevi, tinea versicolor, café au lait macule, port-wine stain, vitiligo
Papule	Solid raised lesion that has distinct borders <1 cm	Acne, molluscum contagiosum, warts, scabies, insect bites
Plaque	Solid, raised, flat-topped lesion >1 cm	
Vesicle	Small fluid filled blister (<0.5 cm)	Chickenpox, herpes, impetigo, friction blisters, pemphigus
Bulla	Large fluid filled blister (>0.5 cm)	
Pustule	Blister containing pus	Acne
Nodule	Raised, solid lesion >1 cm	Neurofibromas, lipomas, tendon xanthoma, rheumatoid nodules
Wheal	Area of oedema of the dermis	Insect bite, drug-induced urticaria
Burrow	Linear or curved elevations of the superficial skin due to infestation of female scabies mite	Scabies
Telangiectasia	Permanent dilatation of superficial blood vessel	Poikiloderma, chronic topical steroid usage
Petechiae	Pinhead-sized, red macules of blood which does not blanch on pressure	Idiopathic thrombocytic purpura, meningococcal septicaemia, trauma, Henoch–Schönlein purpura
Purpura	Larger petechiae	
Ecchymosis	Large extravasation of blood in skin	
Cyst	Cavity lined by epithelium containing fluid, pus, or keratin	Sebaceous cyst, cystic acne
Comedo	Dark, horny keratin and sebaceous plugs within pilosebaceous openings	Acne vulgaris, naevus comedonicus
Secondary lesion		
Scale	Flakes or plates of loose, excess, compacted desquamated layers of stratum corneum	Psoriasis, crusted scabies, ichthyosis vulgaris, pityriasis rosea
Crust	Dried exudate	Acute eczema, ulcers
Lichenification	Thickening of the epidermis with exaggerated skin markings	Neurodermatitis, atopic dermatitis
Excoriation	Abraded skin caused by scratching or rubbing	
Erosion	Partial loss of epidermis which heals without scarring	Pemphigus
Fissure	Linear slit of skin which extends into the dermis	Fissure foot
Ulcer	Necrosis of the epidermis and dermis with or without involvement of the underlying subcutaneous tissue, heals with scarring	
Scar	Permanent changes occurring on skin following damage to the dermis, produced by replacement with fibrous tissue	
Keloid	Excessive scar formation which spreads beyond the original scar line	More commonly seen with dark-skinned people
Atrophy	Thinning of the skin due to shrinkage of epidermis, dermis, or subcutaneous fat	Morphea, discoid lupus erythematosus, atrophic scars

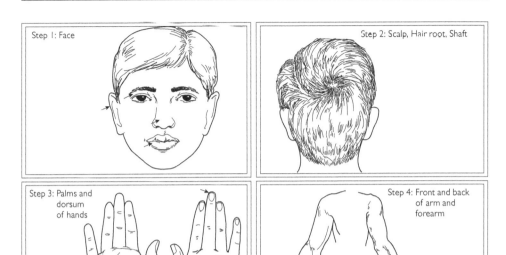

→ Indicates areas which need special attention while examining

Figure 14.4 Step-wise inspection of the skin 1.

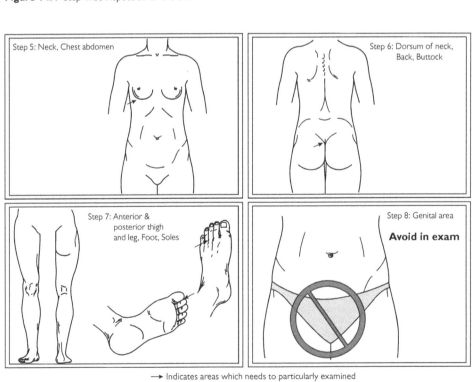

→ Indicates areas which needs to particularly examined

Figure 14.5 Step-wise inspection of the skin 2.

- **Ridges** are raised lines running across the nail and can be transverse (eczema, psoriasis, systemic illness, trauma) or longitudinal (trauma, lichen planus, onychomycosis, and psoriasis).
- Nail plates can **thicken** (fungal infection) or thin out (nail biting).
- **Dystrophic nails** (opalescent, thin, dull, fragile, ridged, and notched) can be seen in 'twenty nail dystrophy' which is characterized by the rough linear ridges on most of the nails of the fingers and toes.
- **Onycholysis** (separation of the nail plate from the proximal nail bed) can be idiopathic or due to trauma, psoriasis, infection, or tumour.
  - Discoloration: diffuse hyperpigmentation of the nail plate is seen in Addison's disease. White nail beds are seen in anaemia, chronic hepatic failure, and chronic renal failure. Blue discoloration of the lunula (the whitish area at the base of the nail) is a sign of Wilson's disease. Yellow discoloration of nail plate can be seen in yellow nail syndrome, onychomycosis, psoriasis, and staining from nail enamel. Purple or black discoloration can be splinter haemorrhages (small areas of bleeding beneath the nails that appear as narrow, reddish-brown lines running along the length of the nail, associated with infective endocarditis) or subungual haematoma (larger collection of blood beneath the nail, caused by trauma).
- Step 2 **cuticle and nail fold**: loss of cuticle can occur in paronychia. Subungual hyperkeratosis (increase in the thickness of the cuticle) can be seen in psoriasis, onychomycosis, and scabies.
- Step 3 **nail shape**: presence of long nails may indicate poor hygiene. Clubbing can be seen in various systemic conditions and is discussed in chapter 5. Though koilonychia (thin, spoon-shaped nail) can be normally seen in infants, it is often occurs due to repeated local injury and in iron deficiency anaemia.
- Step 4 **skin surrounding the nails**: various conditions that may affect the skin adjacent to the nails are viral warts, molluscum contagiosum, corn, and pyogenic granuloma.

Other systems

Relevant systems should be examined depending on the cutaneous finding: arthropathy in psoriasis, growth, abdomen and cataract in Cushing's syndrome, central nervous system in neurocutaneous conditions such as tuberous sclerosis, neurofibromatosis, etc.

Video

Video 14.1 Dr Zengeya will demonstrate examination of the skin. He introduces himself and defines the objective of the examination. He then proceeds to examine not only the skin but also other appendages. At the end he summarizes the findings well and offers a working diagnosis.

Index